# OSTOMY
## DIET COOKBOOK

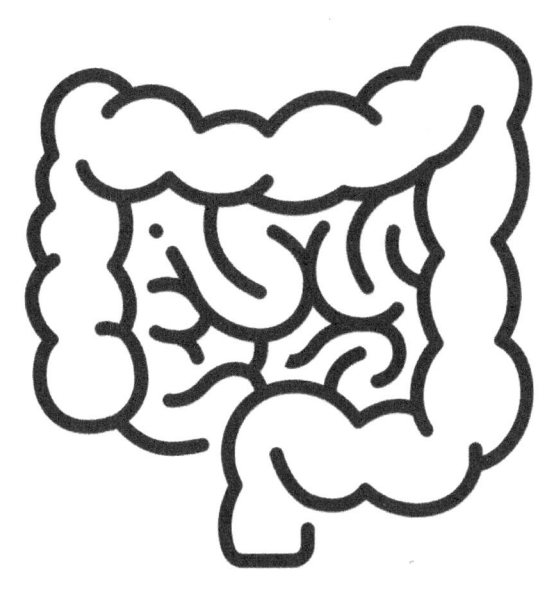

*Everyday Meals for Colostomy and Ileostomy: Delicious Recipes for Health and Comfort*

MISSY RYDER

Copyright © 2025 by Missy Ryder

All rights reserved. No part of this book may be reproduced, stored in a retrieval system, or transmitted in any form or by any means—electronic, mechanical, photocopying, recording, or otherwise—without prior written permission of the publisher, except for brief quotations used in critical reviews or articles. For information, address [Publisher's Contact Information].

## Disclaimer:

The information provided in this book is intended for general guidance and informational purposes only. It is not a substitute for professional medical advice, diagnosis, or treatment. Always seek the advice of your physician or other qualified health provider with any questions you may have regarding a medical condition or treatment. Reliance on any information provided in this book is solely at your own risk.

The author and publisher make no representations or warranties regarding the accuracy, completeness, or suitability of the information contained in this book. In no event shall the author or publisher be liable for any direct, indirect, incidental, or consequential damages arising from the use of or inability to use the information provided in this book.

# TABLE OF CONTENTS

**INTRODUCTION** ........................................................................................................ 8
    THE PURPOSE OF THIS COOKBOOK ........................................................................ 9
    WHO THIS BOOK IS FOR ...................................................................................... 10

**CHAPTER 1** ............................................................................................................ 12

**LIVING WITH A COLOSTOMY** ............................................................................. 12
    TYPES OF COLOSTOMIES ..................................................................................... 12
    WHY MIGHT YOU NEED A COLOSTOMY? ............................................................ 13
    CONDITIONS THAT MAY REQUIRE A PERMANENT COLOSTOMY ......................... 14
    PROCEDURE DETAILS OF A COLOSTOMY ............................................................. 15
    TYPES OF COLOSTOMY OPERATIONS .................................................................. 16
    WHAT NEXT AFTER THE PROCEDURE? ............................................................... 16
    IN THE HOSPITAL ............................................................................................... 17
    AT HOME ............................................................................................................ 18
    WHEN TO CONTACT YOUR HEALTHCARE PROVIDER .......................................... 18
    ADJUSTING TO LIFE WITH A COLOSTOMY .......................................................... 19
    POTENTIAL COMPLICATIONS AFTER LIVING WITH A COLOSTOMY .................... 20
    RECOVERY AND OUTLOOK ................................................................................. 21
    WHAT IS A STOMA? ........................................................................................... 21
    TYPES OF STOMAS ............................................................................................. 21
    WHAT IS THE LIFE EXPECTANCY OF SOMEONE WITH A COLOSTOMY? ............... 23
    THE DIGESTIVE SYSTEM ..................................................................................... 24

**DIET IN COLOSTOMY CARE** ................................................................................ 26
    WHAT IS A COLOSTOMY DIET? .......................................................................... 26
    DIET AFTER COLOSTOMY OR COLECTOMY ........................................................ 26
    ROLE OF DIET IN DIGESTIVE HEALTH ................................................................ 26
    FOODS TO EMBRACE AND AVOID ...................................................................... 28
    AVOIDING COMMON TRIGGERS: GAS, ODOR, AND BLOCKAGES ........................ 29
    HOW TO REINTRODUCE FOODS SAFELY ............................................................ 30

**CHAPTER 2** ............................................................................................................ 32

**BREAKFAST** ........................................................................................................... 32

*Scrambled Eggs with Toast* ................................................................................................ 32
*Egg White Omelet* .............................................................................................................. 33
*Poached Eggs on Toast* ..................................................................................................... 34
*Scrambled Egg Whites with Cheese* ................................................................................ 35
*Whole meal Banana Muffins* ............................................................................................ 36

## CHAPTER 3 ........................................................................................................................ 38

## SOUPS AND STEWS .......................................................................................................... 38

*Cream of Chicken Soup* .................................................................................................... 38
*Chicken Noodle Soup (Without Vegetables)* ................................................................... 39
*Creamy Tomato Soup* ........................................................................................................ 40
*Chicken and Dumpling Soup* ............................................................................................ 41
*Red Lentil Soup* .................................................................................................................. 42
*Minestrone Soup* ................................................................................................................ 43

## CHAPTER 4 ........................................................................................................................ 44

## SALADS AND LIGHT MEALS ............................................................................................ 44

*Tuna Salad on White Bread* .............................................................................................. 44
*Egg Salad Sandwich* .......................................................................................................... 45
*Chicken Caesar Salad (Without Croutons)* ...................................................................... 46
*Tuna Pasta Salad* ............................................................................................................... 47
*Zesty Zucchini Salad* ......................................................................................................... 48
*Roasted Vegetables & Halloumi Salad* ............................................................................ 49

## CHAPTER 5 ........................................................................................................................ 50

## SANDWICHES AND WRAPS ............................................................................................. 50

*Turkey and Swiss Cheese Sandwich* ............................................................................... 50
*Grilled Cheese Sandwich* .................................................................................................. 51
*Turkey and Cream Cheese Roll-ups* ................................................................................ 52
*Grilled Chicken Sandwich* ................................................................................................ 53
*Turkey and Avocado Wrap* ............................................................................................... 54
*Falafel & Pitta Burger* ........................................................................................................ 55

## CHAPTER 6 ........................................................................................................................ 56

## POULTRY DISHES ............................................................................................................. 56

*Simple Chicken Breast with White Rice* .......................................................................... 56

- Baked Chicken Tenders ........................................................................................................... 57
- Chicken Marsala (Without Mushrooms) ................................................................................ 58
- Chicken Alfredo Pasta ............................................................................................................ 59
- Chicken Teriyaki Bowl ............................................................................................................ 60
- Chicken and Rice Casserole ................................................................................................... 61
- One Pot Chicken and Rice ..................................................................................................... 62
- Chicken Curry & Pilaf Rice ..................................................................................................... 63
- Chicken and Vegetable Patties .............................................................................................. 64
- Poached Chicken Breast with Rice Pilaf ................................................................................ 65

## CHAPTER 7 .................................................................................................................................. 66

## BEEF AND PORK DISHES ........................................................................................................... 66

- Lean Turkey Meatloaf ............................................................................................................ 66
- Lean Beef Stir-Fry with White Rice ........................................................................................ 67
- Grilled Pork Chops with Applesauce ..................................................................................... 68
- Lean Ground Beef Patty with White Rice ............................................................................. 69
- Baked Pork Loin with Gravy .................................................................................................. 70
- Lean Beef Stroganoff with Egg Noodles ............................................................................... 71
- Lean Meatballs with White Pasta .......................................................................................... 72
- Lean Beef Pot Roast (without vegetables) ............................................................................ 73
- Lean Beef Lasagna (without ricotta) ..................................................................................... 74
- Grilled Pork Tenderloin with White Rice ............................................................................... 75

## CHAPTER 8 .................................................................................................................................. 76

## SEAFOOD DISHES ....................................................................................................................... 76

- Baked Cod with Lemon Butter .............................................................................................. 76
- Poached Salmon with Dill Sauce ........................................................................................... 77
- Baked Tilapia with Herbs ....................................................................................................... 78
- Steamed White Fish with Lemon .......................................................................................... 79
- Tilapia Fish Cakes ................................................................................................................... 80
- Baked Salmon with Dill Cream Sauce ................................................................................... 81
- Baked Fish Sticks .................................................................................................................... 82
- Tuna Noodle Casserole .......................................................................................................... 83

## CHAPTER 9 .................................................................................................................................. 84

## VEGETARIAN AND VEGAN DISHES ........................................................................................... 84

- Mashed Potato Bowl ......................................................................................................... 84
- Vegetarian Lasagna ......................................................................................................... 85
- Vegan Chili Con Carne ..................................................................................................... 86
- Lentil Nut Roast & Roasted Vegetables ........................................................................... 87
- Tofu, Cashew & Egg Fried Rice ........................................................................................ 88
- Maple-glazed Tofu Roast .................................................................................................. 89
- Penne Pasta ...................................................................................................................... 90
- Cheesy Veggie & Herb Muffins ......................................................................................... 91

## CHAPTER 10 .................................................................................................................. 92

## TURKEY DISHES ............................................................................................................ 92

- Turkey Burger on a White Bun .......................................................................................... 92
- Turkey Tetrazzini ............................................................................................................... 93
- Turkey Meatballs with Quinoa Pasta ................................................................................ 94
- Turkey and Cheese Quesadilla ......................................................................................... 95

## CHAPTER 11 .................................................................................................................. 96

## BAKED GOODS AND DESSERTS ................................................................................. 96

- Bread and Butter Pudding Festive .................................................................................... 96
- Broccoli Gratin Festive ...................................................................................................... 97
- Vanilla Panna Cotta Berry Compote ................................................................................. 98
- Strawberry Cheesecake .................................................................................................... 99
- Banana Cake ................................................................................................................... 100
- Marbled Brownies ........................................................................................................... 101
- French Chocolate Pie ...................................................................................................... 102
- Carrot Cake ..................................................................................................................... 103
- Cream Cheese Frosting .................................................................................................. 104

## CHAPTER 12 ................................................................................................................ 106

## SMOOTHIES AND BEVERAGES ................................................................................. 106

- Creamy Banana Vanilla Shake ........................................................................................ 106
- Smooth Peach Nectar ..................................................................................................... 107
- Mellow Mango Lassi ....................................................................................................... 108
- Black Forest Smoothie .................................................................................................... 109
- Silky Strawberry Yogurt Blend ........................................................................................ 110
- Chilled Honeydew Mint Refresher .................................................................................. 111

*Velvety Chocolate Almond Milk* ........... 112
*Tropical Coconut Pineapple Cooler* ........... 113
*Soothing Chamomile Lemon Tea* ........... 114
*Gentle Ginger Pear Sipper* ........... 115
*Creamy Cantaloupe Cooler* ........... 116

## CHAPTER 13 ........... 118
## MEAL PLAN ........... 118
## CHAPTER 14 ........... 124
## MANAGING COMMON CHALLENGES WITH DIET ........... 124
### Tips for Managing Gas, Odor, and Stool Consistency ........... 124
### What to Do If You Experience Blockages or Discomfort ........... 126
### Strategies for Dining Out and Social Situations ........... 128

## CHAPTER 15 ........... 132
## FAQS AND TROUBLESHOOTING ........... 132
## CONCLUSION ........... 138

# Introduction

Leaving the hospital with a new ostomy is a significant milestone in your journey to recovery. Amidst the heaps of discharge paperwork, you may find yourself staring at what's often called THE LIST—an exhaustive rundown of foods you're advised to avoid. When I first faced this daunting list 14 years ago, it felt like a heavy burden, one that promised a long list of restrictions and limitations on what I could enjoy.

But here's the truth: that list isn't a one-size-fits-all prescription. It's a starting point, not a definitive guide. The reality is what might be a challenge for one person with an ostomy may not be the same for another. My own journey has shown me that while initial guidance can be useful, it's not the final word on what you can or cannot eat.

In the early days at home, I relied on small, bland meals, slowly introducing different foods to see how my body would respond. It was a process of careful observation and adjustment. Foods that caused discomfort or gas before surgery might still have the same effect, and it's important to be aware of that as you begin to expand your diet. The key is to pay attention to how your body reacts and make informed decisions based on your personal experience.

One of the biggest adjustments is learning how to manage your diet with an ostomy. It can be overwhelming to navigate this new reality, especially when you're trying to balance your nutritional needs with comfort and practicality. I found that chewing food thoroughly and staying well-hydrated were crucial. Hydration is a vital concern for those with an ostomy, as it helps maintain overall health and prevent complications.

I always keep a water bottle with me, a simple yet effective way to ensure I'm staying hydrated throughout the day. Over time, you will begin to understand which foods are best suited for your new lifestyle and which ones should be avoided. This book is designed to support you through this process, providing recipes and advice to help you find a diet that works for you.

Adjusting to life with an ostomy can feel daunting, but it doesn't mean you have to give up on enjoying delicious and satisfying meals. It's about discovering what works best for your body and finding joy in your food again. This journey may take time and patience, but with the right guidance and support, you can create a diet that enhances your well-being and suits your personal needs.

## *The Purpose of This Cookbook*

Navigating life with an ostomy or ileostomy can be a complex journey, filled with new routines and adjustments. One of the most significant changes is adapting your diet to ensure it supports your health and comfort while accommodating your new digestive system. This cookbook is designed with that purpose in mind: to offer practical, delicious, and manageable recipes tailored specifically for those living with an ostomy or ileostomy.

**Why This Cookbook Matters**

After surgery, the focus often shifts to learning how to manage your diet to avoid discomfort and complications. You might face challenges like figuring out what foods to include and how to prepare them in a way that suits your new needs. The purpose of this cookbook is to provide clear, practical guidance to make this transition smoother.

1. **Addressing Common Dietary Concerns:** After an ostomy or ileostomy, dietary adjustments are necessary to avoid issues like blockages, excessive gas, or irritation. This cookbook is designed to address these concerns by featuring low-fiber, easy-to-digest recipes that align with the dietary needs of ostomy and ileostomy patients. Each recipe is carefully crafted to be gentle on the digestive system while still offering variety and flavor.

2. **Providing Practical Solutions:** We understand that the early days after surgery can be overwhelming. The recipes in this book offer simple, straightforward solutions to help you manage your diet effectively. From easy-to-prepare meals to tips on what to look for in food, this cookbook aims to reduce the stress and confusion that often accompanies dietary changes post-surgery.

3. **Supporting Nutritional Balance:** Maintaining proper nutrition is crucial, especially when adjusting to a new way of eating. This cookbook ensures that each recipe provides essential nutrients while remaining gentle on your digestive system. By following these recipes, you can feel confident that you're meeting your nutritional needs without compromising your comfort.

4. **Empowering You with Knowledge:** Understanding what works for your body is a key aspect of living well with an ostomy or ileostomy. This cookbook not only provides recipes but also educates you on how different foods impact your digestive health. With this knowledge, you can make informed decisions and personalize your diet to better suit your needs.

5. **Offering Support and Encouragement:** Transitioning to life with an ostomy or ileostomy can be challenging, but you're not alone. This cookbook serves as a companion to guide you through your dietary journey, offering support and encouragement every step of the way. It's designed to help you regain confidence in your food choices and enjoy your meals again.

## *Who This Book Is For*

**Colostomy and Ileostomy Patients**

**Navigating New Dietary Needs:** For individuals adjusting to life with a colostomy or ileostomy, understanding how to adapt your diet is crucial. This cookbook provides you with a variety of low-fiber, easy-to-digest recipes that are designed to fit your new dietary requirements. Each recipe aims to minimize discomfort and support your overall health while helping you explore new, enjoyable foods that align with your digestive needs.

**Building Confidence in Your Diet:** The transition to a new eating routine can be overwhelming. By offering simple, nourishing recipes and practical tips, this cookbook empowers you to take control of your diet, make informed choices, and feel more confident in managing your new digestive system. You'll find guidance on how to reintroduce foods safely and manage any potential dietary challenges.

**Caregivers**

**Supporting Dietary Adjustments:** As a caregiver, understanding the dietary needs of someone with a colostomy or ileostomy is essential. This cookbook equips you with the knowledge and recipes to help prepare meals that are both suitable and satisfying for your loved one. Whether you're planning daily meals or special occasions, the recipes in this book ensure that you can provide nutritious, low-fiber options that cater to their needs.

**Navigating Food Preparation:** Caring for someone with specific dietary requirements can be challenging. This cookbook offers practical advice and easy-to-follow recipes to make meal preparation more manageable. You'll find guidance on ingredient selection and cooking techniques that accommodate dietary restrictions while still delivering flavorful and enjoyable meals.

**Family Members**

**Understanding Dietary Needs:** Family members play a crucial role in supporting their loved ones through dietary adjustments. This cookbook helps you understand what foods are beneficial and why, providing insight into how dietary choices can impact the comfort and health of a person with a colostomy or ileostomy. By learning about suitable foods and meal planning, you can offer meaningful support and contribute to their well-being.

**Creating Inclusive Meals:** Involving the entire family in meal planning and preparation can foster a supportive environment and make mealtimes more enjoyable. This cookbook includes recipes that are easy to prepare and cater to specific dietary needs, making it easier to create meals that everyone can enjoy together, without the need for separate, specialized dishes.

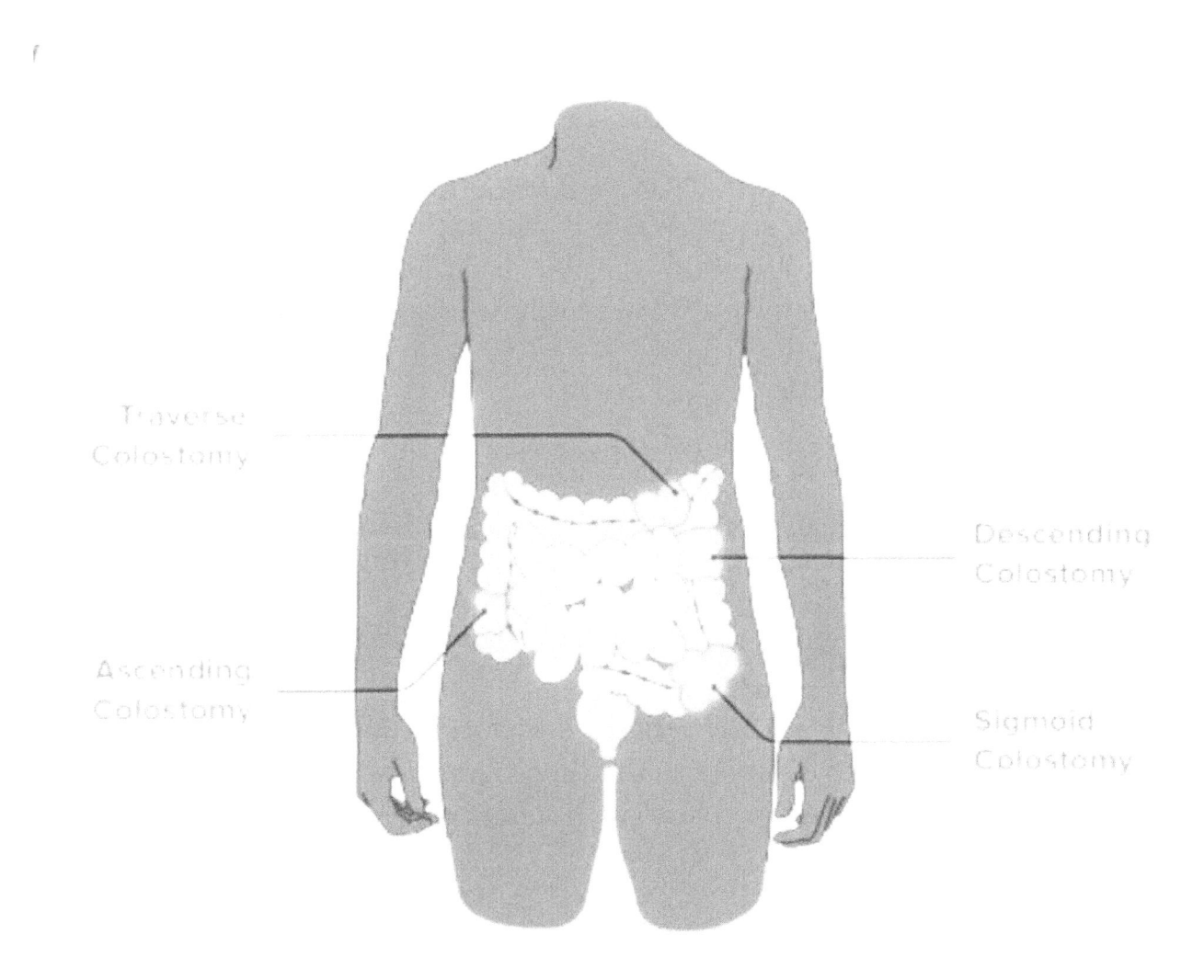

# Chapter 1

# Living with a Colostomy

A colostomy is a surgical procedure that creates an opening in the abdomen for the colon (large intestine). This opening, known as a stoma, allows waste (stool) to exit the body into a bag attached to the abdomen. Colostomies can be temporary, to allow the bowel time to heal, or permanent, often necessary after bowel surgery or injury.

In a permanent colostomy, the end of the colon is brought through the abdominal wall and attached to the skin, forming a stoma. Waste is then expelled through the stoma into a colostomy bag. Temporary colostomies, on the other hand, involve bringing a portion of the colon to the surface of the abdomen, and can usually be reversed once healing is complete.

## *Types of Colostomies*

1. **Temporary Colostomy**

    A temporary colostomy is used to divert waste away from a healing section of the bowel. After the bowel has healed, the colostomy can often be reversed, allowing normal bowel function to resume.

2. **Permanent Colostomy**

    A permanent colostomy is typically performed when a portion of the rectum or colon is diseased, such as in cases of cancer. In this procedure, the affected part of the colon is removed or bypassed, and the colostomy becomes a permanent solution for waste elimination.

3. **Transverse Colostomy**

    Transverse colostomies are common and occur in the upper abdomen. They divert waste away from the descending colon and are generally temporary. There are two main types:

    - **Loop Transverse Colostomy:** Creates two openings in the stoma—one for waste and another for mucus, a normal byproduct of digestion.

- **Double-Barrel Transverse Colostomy:** Divides the bowel into two sections, each with its own stoma—one for stool and one for mucus.

Transverse colostomies are often accompanied by a lightweight, drainable pouch to collect waste and protect the skin, which can be easily concealed under clothing.

4. **Ascending Colostomy**

    An ascending colostomy is located on the right side of the abdomen, where only a small section of the colon remains active. The output is typically liquid and rich in digestive enzymes, necessitating the constant use of a drainable pouch. These colostomies are less common today, with ileostomies often preferred.

5. **Descending and Sigmoid Colostomies**

    - **Descending Colostomy:** Positioned in the descending colon on the lower left side of the abdomen, this colostomy generally produces more solid waste that can often be regulated.

    - **Sigmoid Colostomy:** Located on the sigmoid colon, slightly lower than a descending colostomy, this type allows the most normal bowel function, with regular, formed stool output.

## *Why Might You Need a Colostomy?*

A colostomy may be necessary for various medical conditions that affect the colon or rectum. Reasons for undergoing a colostomy include:

- **Birth Defects:** Conditions like an imperforate anus, where the anal opening is blocked or missing, may require a colostomy.

- **Diverticular Disease:** Diverticula are small pouches in the colon that can become infected (diverticulitis) or cause significant bleeding, necessitating bowel surgery.

- **Inflammatory Bowel Disease (IBD):** Severe inflammation, such as from Crohn's disease or ulcerative colitis, can require a colostomy.

- **Injury to the Colon or Rectum:** Trauma or severe injury may necessitate a colostomy to allow the area to heal.

- **Bowel Obstruction:** Partial or complete blockage of the intestines can make a colostomy necessary to bypass the affected section.

- **Colorectal Cancer:** Surgery for rectal or colon cancer may involve creating a colostomy, especially if large portions of the colon or rectum are removed.

- **Serious Infections:** Severe infections like diverticulitis or abscesses may require diverting waste to allow healing.

- **Anal Fistulas:** These abnormal connections between the anus and skin or another organ may necessitate a colostomy.

- **Partial Colectomies:** When parts of the colon are surgically removed, a colostomy may be used temporarily until the bowel can be reattached.

## *Conditions That May Require a Permanent Colostomy*

- **Incurable Fecal Incontinence:** When bowel control cannot be restored, a permanent colostomy may be necessary.

- **Advanced Colorectal Cancer:** Surgery to remove the rectum or anus due to cancer often results in a permanent colostomy.

- **Permanent Removal of the Rectum or Anus:** This may be required if the rectal muscles fail, or if cancer has significantly spread.

**What's the Difference Between a Colostomy and an Ileostomy?**

The main difference between a colostomy and an ileostomy lies in which part of the intestines is diverted to the abdominal wall. The colon (large intestine) is involved in a colostomy, while the ileum (part of the small intestine) is involved in an ileostomy. Normally, waste travels from the ileum into the colon, where it is formed into solid stool. However, if the colon is removed or inactive, this process is disrupted.

In an ileostomy, the ileum is redirected to a stoma on the abdomen. Waste is expelled in liquid form from the small intestine into an ostomy bag attached to the stoma. Like a colostomy, an ileostomy can be temporary or permanent, depending on the underlying condition. In some cases, when the colon is no longer functional, surgeons may create an internal "ileal pouch" as a substitute, which allows for the closure of the stoma.

**How Common is Ostomy Surgery?**

Ostomy surgery is quite common, with approximately 100,000 people in the United States undergoing the procedure each year. Around 1 in 500 Americans, or up to 1 million people, live with an ostomy and often refer to themselves as "ostomates." Due to its prevalence, there is a wide range of specialized products available, including various types of ostomy bags, as well as underwear and swimwear designed to help ostomates manage their condition discreetly. Ostomy support groups are also widely available to provide community and assistance.

## *Procedure Details of a Colostomy*

**What Happens Before a Colostomy?**

A colostomy is a significant surgical procedure that requires careful preparation.

**Before the Surgery:** You will have a pre-operation assessment meeting with your surgeon, where they will explain the procedure, potential risks, and the lifestyle changes you may need to make afterward. This meeting also includes discussing pain management options before you sign your consent forms. A nurse will take a blood sample to ensure you are fit for surgery, and you may also undergo an EKG test to check your heart's health.

**On the Day of the Surgery:** You will need to refrain from eating or drinking for six hours before the surgery. In some cases, you may be instructed to use an enema or bowel prep like that used before a colonoscopy, which you will complete at home. Upon arrival at the hospital, you will change into a hospital gown and wait in a pre-op room. Once in the operating room, you will be given anesthesia to prepare you for surgery.

**What Happens During the Colostomy Procedure?**

Colostomies can be performed using either laparoscopic surgery or open surgery:

**Laparoscopic Surgery:**

This modern, minimally invasive technique uses a small, lighted camera called a laparoscope. Your surgeon makes a small incision in your abdomen to insert the laparoscope, which projects images of your abdominal organs onto a screen. The surgery is completed using additional small incisions, allowing the surgeon to access your organs. Laparoscopic surgery often results in fewer complications, reduced pain, and a quicker recovery. However, some complex cases may require converting to open surgery during the procedure.

**Open Surgery:**

Open surgery involves a single, longer incision to access the abdominal cavity. This traditional approach provides better access to the abdominal organs, which can be necessary for certain conditions. However, it is a major surgery with a longer recovery period compared to laparoscopic surgery. The decision between open and laparoscopic surgery depends on the specific condition being treated and any additional procedures that may be required during the colostomy. Typically, you will be informed in advance about the type of surgery you will undergo, allowing you to plan accordingly.

## *Types of Colostomy Operations*

There are two main types of colostomy surgeries commonly performed:

**Loop Colostomy**

A loop colostomy is usually chosen when the colostomy is intended to be temporary, as it is easier to reverse. During this procedure, the surgeon selects the section of the bowel that will form the colostomy and pulls it through an incision in the abdomen as a loop. The loop is then cut, and the two ends are positioned side by side in the abdominal opening, creating a stoma with two openings. One opening allows stool to pass from the active part of the bowel, while the other, connected to the inactive part of the bowel, discharges mucus that exits through the anus.

**End Colostomy**

An end colostomy is often performed when the colostomy is likely to be permanent. In this procedure, after the bowel is divided, the active end is stitched to the abdominal wall to form the stoma, while the inactive end is sealed. The stoma serves as the exit point for stool, and if the anus is still intact, mucus may be discharged through the anus instead of a second stoma.

## *What Next After the Procedure?*

After a colostomy, the section of your colon that was affected will influence your recovery and the characteristics of your stoma output.

**Ascending Colostomy**

The ascending colon is the first section of the large intestine, located on the right side of the abdomen. In an ascending colostomy, a small portion of the colon remains functional. Waste from the small intestine entering this part is still liquid and contains digestive enzymes. This liquid output passes through the stoma, requiring special care to prevent skin irritation and manage leakage due to the presence of these enzymes.

**Transverse Colostomy**

The transverse colon is the middle section of the colon, running horizontally across the abdomen. Transverse colostomies are often performed to allow the lower bowel to rest or to bypass it permanently. The stool from this type of colostomy will be semi-solid with fewer digestive enzymes than an ascending colostomy but still different from normal stool. The stoma may be positioned higher on the abdomen, which can pose challenges in concealing it under clothing.

**Descending and Sigmoid Colostomies**

The descending and sigmoid colons are located on the left side of the abdomen. A colostomy in these sections retains most of the colon's function, resulting in more formed stool that is less irritating to the skin. With these types, bowel movements may occur more predictably, allowing some individuals to manage their output more effectively.

## *In the Hospital*

A colostomy typically requires a hospital stay of 3 to 7 days, longer if performed as an emergency. During your stay, you'll learn how to care for your colostomy and use the pouch that collects stool. Nurses will guide you on cleaning your stoma daily with warm water, gently patting or air drying the area.

You'll be introduced to various types of pouches made from odor-resistant materials, particularly important for those with ascending or transverse colostomies who need to always wear a drainable pouch. Those with descending or sigmoid colostomies might predict bowel movements and wear pouches only as needed or learn to irrigate their stoma to control bowel activity.

Before discharge, consult with an ostomy nurse or specialist to determine the best equipment for your needs. Factors like stoma length, abdominal shape, scars, folds, and your overall body composition will influence your choice.

If the rectum and anus were removed, resulting in a posterior wound, you'll learn to care for it with dressings, pads, and possibly sitz baths (warm, shallow soaks). Your healthcare provider will give you specific instructions for wound care, and you should contact them if you encounter any complications.

## At Home

The skin around your stoma should resemble the healthy skin on the rest of your abdomen, but exposure to stool, especially loose stool, can lead to irritation. Here are some tips to protect your skin:

1. **Ensure Proper Fit:** Make sure your pouch and skin barrier opening are the correct size to prevent leaks.
2. **Change Regularly:** Replace the pouch when it is about one-third full to avoid leakage and skin irritation. Don't wait for itching or burning to occur.
3. **Gentle Removal:** Remove the pouching system carefully, pushing the skin away from the adhesive rather than pulling.
4. **Use Barrier Creams:** Apply barrier creams if irritation develops, even with preventive measures.

## When to Contact Your Healthcare Provider

Notify your healthcare provider if you experience any of the following symptoms:

- Severe cramps lasting more than two hours
- Blockage or collapse of the stoma
- Excessive bleeding from the stoma or blood in the pouch (Note: consuming beets can cause red discoloration in stool)
- Significant injury or cut to the stoma
- Persistent skin irritation
- Continuous nausea or vomiting
- Unusual odor lasting more than a week
- Changes in stoma size or color
- Blocked or protruding stoma
- Watery stool for more than five hours
- Frequent pouch leakage, making it difficult to keep it on for two to three days
- Any other concerning symptoms

**Pouching Tips**

Empty your pouch when it is one-third to half full and change it before it starts to leak. Pouch systems vary in durability, with some needing replacement daily and others lasting up to a week. Consult your healthcare team about financial resources that may help cover the costs of colostomy supplies.

## *Adjusting to Life with a Colostomy*

Living with a colostomy is a significant adjustment. Although you may feel the pouch against your skin, it is not visible to others. You do not have to explain your colostomy to anyone unless you choose to share.

Some individuals and their families may experience feelings of depression, anxiety, or self-esteem issues due to the changes a colostomy brings. Seek mental health support if you or your loved ones are struggling with the adjustment. A simple way to explain your condition is to mention you had abdominal surgery. Consider joining a support group for those with colostomies. Your healthcare team or ostomy nurse can connect you with these valuable resources.

**What Are the Risks of the Procedure?**

Undergoing a colostomy is a major life change, but the surgical procedure itself is relatively straightforward. The surgery is performed under general anesthesia, so you will be asleep and will not feel any pain. It can be done as open surgery with one large incision or laparoscopically with several smaller incisions.

**Risks associated with anesthesia include:**

- Breathing problems
- Adverse reactions to medications

**Surgical risks specific to a colostomy include:**

- Bleeding
- Damage to nearby organs
- Infection

**Post-surgery risks include:**

- Narrowing of the colostomy opening

- Intestinal blockage from scar tissue
- Skin irritation
- Wound dehiscence (opening of the wound)
- Hernia development at the incision site

## *Potential Complications After Living with a Colostomy*

Even after successful surgery, there are possible complications that can arise while living with a colostomy:

- **Skin irritation:** This is the most common issue and usually occurs from contact with stool, especially if it's acidic or liquid. Skin irritation can often be resolved with a better-fitting colostomy bag.

- **Bowel obstructions:** These can result from scar tissue or paralytic ileus (a slowing of the intestines), causing a blockage. Home remedies for constipation may help in managing this.

- **Stoma retraction or prolapse:** A retracted stoma sits below the skin's surface, while a prolapsed stoma extends too far outward. Both conditions can make it difficult to secure the colostomy bag. In severe cases, a surgical revision may be necessary.

- **Parastomal hernia:** This occurs when bowel loops bulge through weakened abdominal muscles near the stoma, forming a noticeable bulge that can grow and potentially block the stoma's output. Preventative measures will be discussed with your colostomy nurse.

## *Recovery and Outlook*

**What Is the Recovery Time from a Colostomy?**

Recovery in the hospital typically lasts between three to seven days. During this time, you will:

- **Gradually resume eating:** Initially, you will be placed on a clear liquid diet, followed by a full liquid or soft diet before transitioning back to solid foods.

- **Learn colostomy care:** A wound ostomy continence nurse (WOCN) will guide you on how to care for your stoma and manage your colostomy bag.

- **Wean off pain medications:** You will gradually reduce your pain medications and may be given a short-term prescription to take home.

- **Heal and regulate bowel movements:** It may take several days post-surgery before your first bowel movement, and your bowel function will gradually stabilize as you recover.

## *What Is a Stoma?*

The terms 'stoma' and 'ostomy' are often used interchangeably, but they refer to different aspects of the procedure. A stoma is a surgically created opening on the abdomen's surface that diverts the flow of feces or urine. Individuals who have undergone stoma surgery are sometimes referred to as 'ostomates.'

Initially, your stoma may appear bruised, red, and swollen. This appearance will gradually improve over the following weeks as it shrinks and becomes a soft red or pink color. Since the stoma is an internal part of your intestines exposed on the outside, it will generally be round. Its appearance can vary among individuals; it may protrude slightly or lie flat against the skin.

## *Types of Stomas*

There are three main types of stomas, each serving a different purpose based on its location and function:

**Colostomy**
A colostomy involves creating an opening from the colon (large intestine). During this procedure, a portion of the colon is brought through an incision in the abdomen and secured to the surface. This opening is typically located on the left side of the abdomen.

The output from a colostomy can vary, but it usually functions about 1 to 3 times a day, with output that tends to be more solid and like traditional stool.

**Ileostomy**

An ileostomy involves creating an opening from the small intestine, specifically the ileum. In this procedure, a section of the small intestine is brought through the abdomen and secured on the outside. This type of stoma is usually positioned on the right side of the abdomen. Ileostomy output is generally looser compared to a colostomy and may require the ileostomy bag to be emptied 3 to 6 times a day.

**Urostomy**

A urostomy, also known as an ileal conduit, is an opening for urine diversion. It involves taking a segment of the small intestine and attaching the ureters to it to form a passageway for urine. The end of this segment is brought out through the abdomen to create the urostomy. Usually, the bladder is removed, although this depends on the specific surgery. The urostomy is typically located on the right side of the abdomen and features a small spout for urine to exit. The urostomy bag often includes a bung or tap for regular drainage into the toilet.

**What Does It Feel Like to Have a Stoma?**

During the initial healing phase after a colostomy, you might experience some discomfort around the wound. Over-the-counter pain relievers can help manage this pain temporarily. The stoma itself, being the end of your intestine, lacks nerve endings and does not produce any sensation. Once the surrounding surgical wound heals, you should not feel the stoma.

Emotionally, having a stoma can bring up a range of feelings. You may worry about how others will react or feel about your stoma. Speaking with your ostomy nurse can be helpful in addressing these concerns. They can provide support and connect you with others who have similar experiences.

**Can You Still Poop with a Colostomy Bag?**

Having a colostomy changes how you pass stool. Right after surgery, your anus may continue to expel any residual waste, but new stool will exit through the stoma. Although you may feel bowel movements, you will not have control over them as you did before. Unlike the anus, the stoma lacks muscles to allow for voluntary closure, so stool will pass through it involuntarily.

Some individuals with a removed colon might experience phantom urges for bowel movements, like phantom limb sensations. These urges often diminish if they sit on the toilet as they used to. If your anus remains intact and you don't have a separate stoma for anal discharge, you will still pass occasional mucus through your anus. This mucus helps to lubricate and protect the skin as part of the inactive colon's regular function.

**Will I Always Have to Wear a Colostomy Bag?**

Many people opt to wear a colostomy bag continuously to manage stool output. Modern colostomy bags are designed to be discreet and can be worn under most clothing. However, if you have a descending or sigmoid colostomy and a significant portion of your colon remains functional, you might be able to predict bowel movements and wear the pouch only during these times. Some individuals may also practice colostomy irrigation, a process that involves flushing the bowel with water to induce regular movements and potentially go without a bag between irrigations.

## *What Is the Life Expectancy of Someone with a Colostomy?*

A colostomy is often performed for life-threatening conditions, and the procedure itself aims to improve the patient's overall prognosis. While a colostomy can enhance quality of life, the life expectancy of an individual depends on various factors beyond the surgery, such as the underlying condition and overall health. The average age for colostomy patients is around 70, and other health issues may also affect life expectancy.

**When Can I Have a Colostomy Reversal?**

The timing for a colostomy reversal depends on several factors, including:

- **The reason for your colostomy:** The underlying condition that necessitated the colostomy will influence the possibility and timing of a reversal.
- **Your post-surgery health:** Your overall health and recovery status will be evaluated.
- **Your ability to undergo additional surgery:** Your general health and readiness for another surgical procedure are crucial.

If your colostomy was meant to be temporary, you can discuss the possibility of reversal with your doctor during follow-up appointments. Your doctor will assess your condition and determine the appropriate time for the reversal surgery, which could range from a few months to a year after the initial procedure, or even longer in some cases. There is no set timeframe for a reversal; the decision is based on your health and recovery.

**When to Contact Your Doctor**

You should reach out to your healthcare provider or ostomy nurse if you experience:

- Persistent constipation or diarrhea
- Ongoing nausea or vomiting
- Presence of blood in your stool
- Noticeable changes in your stoma's size or color
- Unusual or foul odors from your stoma
- Any blockage in your stoma

## *The Digestive System*

A colostomy does not alter the fundamental functioning of your digestive system. After you chew and swallow food, it travels down the esophagus into your stomach. From the stomach, it moves into the small intestine and then into the large intestine (colon). The indigestible remnants are eventually expelled from the rectum through the anus as stool.

As stool moves through the upper colon, it remains loose and liquid. Water is absorbed as it travels further, causing the stool to become firmer by the time it reaches the rectum. The colon is divided into sections:

- **Ascending Colon:** Located on the right side of the body, where the stool is more liquid, acidic, and contains digestive enzymes.
- **Transverse Colon:** Extends across the upper abdomen, where stool is less liquid and less acidic.
- **Descending and Sigmoid Colon:** Descend on the left side and curve towards the rectum. Here, the stool becomes progressively firmer and contains fewer digestive enzymes.

The location of the colostomy will affect how irritating the stool may be to the skin. More liquid and acidic stool will necessitate greater care to protect your abdominal skin.

**How to Care for Yourself at Home**

**Activity:**

- **Rest as Needed:** Ensure you get plenty of sleep to aid in your recovery.
- **Daily Walking:** Begin with short walks and gradually increase the distance as you feel able. Walking helps improve circulation and reduces the risk of pneumonia.
- **Avoid Strenuous Activities:** Refrain from engaging in heavy exercises such as biking, jogging, weightlifting, or aerobic workouts until cleared by your doctor.
- **Limit Lifting:** For at least 6 weeks, avoid lifting heavy items such as grocery bags, briefcases, pet food, or vacuum cleaners. This also includes heavy children.
- **Driving:** Consult your doctor to determine when it's safe for you to resume driving.
- **Work Absence:** You may need to take up to 6 weeks off from work, depending on your job and recovery progress.
- **Bathing:** You can bathe or shower as usual, with or without your colostomy bag.
- **Sexual Activity:** Ask your doctor for guidance on when it is safe to resume sexual activity.

# Diet in Colostomy Care

## *What is a Colostomy Diet?*

A colostomy diet refers to the nutritional guidelines you follow undergoing colostomy surgery. Initially, you'll start with a clear liquid diet for several days, which includes water, broth, and plain gelatin. This helps your digestive system begin to recover.

Following the clear liquid phase, you will gradually transition to a high-protein, low-residue diet. This diet minimizes the amount of undigested material left in your gut, consisting of bland, easy-to-digest foods to avoid gastrointestinal discomfort. Adhering to this diet is crucial for a smooth recovery. Once you're sufficiently healed, you can reintroduce your regular foods under the guidance of your doctor or dietitian.

## *Diet After Colostomy or Colectomy*

- **Initial Phase:** Depending on the type of surgery, you may be given only intravenous (IV) fluids for 2 to 3 days to allow your colon to heal. Clear liquids like soup broth and juices (e.g., apple, grape, cranberry) can be introduced once you're able to tolerate them.

- **Hydration:** Ensure you drink plenty of fluids (8 to 10 cups daily) to stay hydrated. Increase your fluid intake in hot weather or to replace fluids lost due to diarrhea.

- **Transition to Solid Foods:** Begin with easy-to-digest foods such as white toast, white rice, applesauce, and chicken breast. Gradually, you can return to your regular diet as tolerated.

- **Managing Odors and Gas:** If you have a colostomy, consider avoiding foods that may cause odors or gas, which could cause the colostomy bag to inflate and become more difficult to manage.

## *Role of Diet in Digestive Health*

Diet plays a crucial role in maintaining and improving digestive health. A balanced and nutritious diet can support digestive functions, prevent disorders, and promote overall well-being. Here's how diet impacts digestive health:

## 1. Supporting Digestive Function

- **Fiber:** Dietary fiber, found in fruits, vegetables, whole grains, and legumes, helps regulate bowel movements by adding bulk to the stool and facilitating its passage through the digestive tract. It can prevent constipation and support regularity.

- **Hydration:** Drinking adequate water helps keep the digestive system running smoothly, preventing dehydration, which can lead to constipation. Proper hydration also supports the absorption of nutrients and the elimination of waste.

- **Healthy Fats:** Sources of healthy fats, like avocados, nuts, and olive oil, can help with the absorption of fat-soluble vitamins (A, D, E, K) and provide essential fatty acids that support the health of the digestive tract.

## 2. Preventing Digestive Disorders

- **Probiotics:** Consuming foods rich in probiotics, such as yogurt, kefir, and fermented vegetables, can help maintain a healthy balance of gut bacteria. Probiotics support digestion, enhance nutrient absorption, and may prevent gastrointestinal disorders like irritable bowel syndrome (IBS) and inflammatory bowel disease (IBD).

- **Limiting Processed Foods:** Reducing the intake of highly processed foods, which can be high in sugars, unhealthy fats, and additives, can prevent issues such as bloating, gas, and digestive discomfort. Opt for whole, unprocessed foods whenever possible.

## 3. Managing Digestive Conditions

- **Low-FODMAP Diet:** For individuals with IBS, a low-FODMAP diet, which restricts certain fermentable carbohydrates, can help reduce symptoms such as bloating, gas, and abdominal pain.

- **Gluten-Free Diet:** Those with celiac disease or gluten sensitivity should avoid gluten-containing foods to prevent digestive distress and inflammation in the intestines.

## 4. Promoting Overall Digestive Health

- **Balanced Meals:** Eating a balanced diet with a variety of nutrients helps maintain overall digestive health. Incorporate a mix of proteins, healthy fats, and carbohydrates, and focus on portion control to prevent overeating and digestive strain.

- **Mindful Eating:** Eating slowly and chewing food thoroughly can aid digestion. Avoid overeating and manage portion sizes to reduce the risk of digestive issues such as acid reflux or indigestion.

## *Foods to Embrace and Avoid*

**Foods to Include:**

- Non-fat or low-fat skim milk
- Lactose-free dairy products
- Yogurt
- Cheese
- Lean animal proteins
- Small amounts of nut butter or nuts
- Low-fiber carbohydrates, such as white pasta or bread
- Well-cooked vegetables without skin
- Lettuce
- Pulp-free fruit juice.
- Peeled or canned fruit
- The flesh of thick-skinned fruits like watermelon or honeydew melon

**Bland Foods:**

- Broth
- Tofu
- White pasta
- Beets
- Beans
- Spinach
- Carrots
- Eggs
- Lean proteins
- Fruit juice

**Liquid Diet:**

- Clear fruit juices (no pulp)
- Broth
- Sports drinks
- Gelatin
- Water
- Decaffeinated tea or coffee

**Foods to Avoid:**

- High-fiber foods
- Carbonated beverages
- High-fat or fried foods
- Raw fruits with skin
- Raw vegetables
- Whole grains
- Fried poultry and fish
- Legumes
- High-fat dairy products
- Spicy foods

**Eating Guidelines:**

- **Eat Slowly and Chew Thoroughly:** Take your time with each meal, chewing your food well to aid digestion. Aim to chew everything until it's liquid in your mouth.
- **Opt for Small, Frequent Meals:** Instead of three large meals, aim for six small meals throughout the day.
- **Stay Hydrated:** Drink 8 to 10 cups (approximately 2 liters) of liquids daily.
- **Focus on Bland, Low-Fiber Foods:** Stick to bland and low-fiber foods to aid your recovery.
- **Reintroduce Foods Gradually:** When reintroducing foods into your diet, add them one at a time to monitor how your body reacts.

## *Avoiding Common Triggers: Gas, Odor, and Blockages*

**Managing Gas:**

- **Avoid Gas-Producing Foods:** Common culprits include beans, lentils, carbonated drinks, and certain vegetables like broccoli and cabbage.
- **Eat Slowly:** Swallowing air while eating can contribute to gas. Take your time and chew thoroughly.
- **Keep a Food Diary:** Track which foods seem to cause gas and adjust your diet accordingly.

**Reducing Odor:**

- **Limit Odor-Causing Foods:** Foods like garlic, onions, and certain spices can increase odor. Reduce or avoid these in your diet.

- **Stay Hydrated:** Drinking plenty of water can help dilute odors.
- **Use Odor-Reducing Products:** Consider using deodorizing products designed for colostomy bags or adding odor-neutralizing tablets to your bag.

**Preventing Blockages:**

- **Avoid High-Fiber Foods:** Foods like whole grains, nuts, and seeds can cause blockages. Opt for lower-fiber alternatives.
- **Chew Food Thoroughly:** Ensure food is well-chewed to prevent large pieces from causing blockages.
- **Eat Small Portions:** Large meals can increase the risk of blockages. Try smaller, more frequent meals.

**General Tips:**

- **Monitor Your Reactions:** Pay attention to how different foods affect your colostomy and adjust as needed.
- **Consult with a Dietitian:** A dietitian can help create a meal plan tailored to your needs and help manage any dietary issues.
- **Stay in Touch with Your Healthcare Team:** Regular check-ins with your healthcare provider can help address any persistent issues and adjust your care plan.

## *How to Reintroduce Foods Safely*

**1. Start Slowly:**

- **Introduce One Food at a Time:** Reintroduce one new food every few days to monitor its effects. This helps identify any adverse reactions or sensitivities.
- **Begin with Small Portions:** Start with a small amount of the new food to gauge how well your digestive system tolerates it.

**2. Opt for Gentle Foods:**

- **Choose Low-Fiber Options:** Begin with foods that are easy to digest and less likely to cause issues, such as well-cooked vegetables and lean proteins.

- **Avoid High-Fiber or Hard-to-Digest Foods Initially:** Foods like raw vegetables, whole grains, and nuts should be reintroduced later, after you've adjusted to other foods.

3. **Observe and Record Reactions:**

    - **Keep a Food Diary:** Track what you eat and note any symptoms or reactions. This can help you pinpoint which foods are well-tolerated and which ones may cause problems.
    - **Watch for Symptoms:** Pay attention to any signs of discomfort, gas, bloating, or blockages.

4. **Adjust Based on Tolerance:**

    - **Increase Portion Sizes Gradually:** If a new food is well-tolerated, you can slowly increase the portion size.
    - **Modify Cooking Methods:** Opt for cooking methods that make foods easier to digest, such as steaming or baking, rather than frying.

5. **Incorporate Foods in a Balanced Way:**

    - **Add a Variety of Foods:** As you reintroduce foods, aim for a balanced diet that includes proteins, carbohydrates, and healthy fats.
    - **Ensure Nutritional Balance:** Include a range of nutrients to maintain overall health and well-being.

6. **Communicate with Your Healthcare Team:**

    - **Report Any Issues:** Inform your healthcare provider of any difficulties or concerns with reintroducing foods. They can offer additional guidance and support.

# Chapter 2

# Breakfast

## Scrambled Eggs with Toast

**Prep Time:** 5 minutes | **Cooking Time:** 5 minutes | **Total Time:** 10 minutes | **Serving:** 1 | **Cooking Difficulty:** Easy

Ingredients:

- 2 large eggs
- 1 tablespoon milk (lactose-free if needed)
- 1 teaspoon butter or oil
- 1 slice white bread, toasted
- Salt and pepper, to taste

Instructions:

1. In a bowl, whisk together the eggs and milk until well combined.
2. Heat the butter or oil in a non-stick skillet over medium heat.
3. Pour the egg mixture into the skillet. Cook, stirring gently, until the eggs are scrambled and cooked through.
4. Season with salt and pepper to taste.
5. Serve the scrambled eggs on top of the toasted white bread.

**Nutritional Value:** Calories: 300 | Fat: 20g | Saturated Fat: 10g | Cholesterol: 370mg | Sodium: 500mg | Carbohydrate: 23g | Fiber: 1g | Added Sugar: 0g | Protein: 15g | Calcium: 180mg | Potassium: 300mg | Phosphorus: 250mg | Iron: 2mg | Vitamin D: 10% DV

# Egg White Omelet

**Prep Time:** 5 minutes | **Cooking Time:** 10 minutes | **Total Time:** 15 minutes | **Serving:** 1 | **Cooking Difficulty:** Easy

Ingredients:

- 3 egg whites
- 1 tablespoon milk (lactose-free if needed)
- 1 teaspoon olive oil
- 1/4 cup shredded low-fat cheese
- Salt and pepper, to taste

Instructions:

1. In a bowl, whisk together the egg whites and milk.
2. Heat the olive oil in a non-stick skillet over medium heat.
3. Pour the egg white mixture into the skillet. Cook until the edges start to set.
4. Sprinkle the shredded cheese over one half of the omelet.
5. Fold the omelet in half and cook until fully set.
6. Season with salt and pepper to taste.

**Nutritional Value:** Calories: 180 | Fat: 8g | Saturated Fat: 1g | Cholesterol: 0mg | Sodium: 300mg | Carbohydrate: 2g | Fiber: 0g | Added Sugar: 0g | Protein: 20g | Calcium: 200mg | Potassium: 250mg | Phosphorus: 150mg | Iron: 1mg | Vitamin D: 0% DV

# Poached Eggs on Toast

**Prep Time:** 5 minutes | **Cooking Time:** 5 minutes | **Total Time:** 10 minutes | **Serving:** 1 | **Cooking Difficulty:** Easy

**Ingredients:**

- 2 large eggs
- 1 slice white bread, toasted
- 1 teaspoon vinegar
- Salt and pepper, to taste

**Instructions:**

1. Fill a saucepan with water and add vinegar. Bring to a simmer.
2. Crack each egg into a small cup and gently slide into the simmering water.
3. Cook for about 3-4 minutes, or until the whites are set and the yolks are still runny.
4. Carefully remove the eggs with a slotted spoon and place them on the toasted white bread.
5. Season with salt and pepper to taste.

**Nutritional Value:** Calories: 250 | Fat: 16g | Saturated Fat: 6g | Cholesterol: 370mg | Sodium: 250mg | Carbohydrate: 23g | Fiber: 1g | Added Sugar: 0g | Protein: 14g | Calcium: 180mg | Potassium: 270mg | Phosphorus: 200mg | Iron: 2mg | Vitamin D: 10% DV

# Scrambled Egg Whites with Cheese

**Prep Time:** 5 minutes | **Cooking Time:** 5 minutes | **Total Time:** 10 minutes | **Serving:** 1 | **Cooking Difficulty:** Easy

**Ingredients:**

- 4 egg whites
- 1 tablespoon milk (lactose-free if needed)
- 1 teaspoon butter or oil
- 1/4 cup shredded low-fat cheese
- Salt and pepper, to taste

**Instructions:**

1. In a bowl, whisk together the egg whites and milk.
2. Heat the butter or oil in a non-stick skillet over medium heat.
3. Pour the egg white mixture into the skillet. Cook, stirring gently, until the egg whites are scrambled and cooked through.
4. Sprinkle the shredded cheese on top and stir until melted.
5. Season with salt and pepper to taste.

**Nutritional Value:** Calories: 200 | Fat: 10g | Saturated Fat: 5g | Cholesterol: 0mg | Sodium: 400mg | Carbohydrate: 2g | Fiber: 0g | Added Sugar: 0g | Protein: 20g | Calcium: 200mg | Potassium: 300mg | Phosphorus: 150mg | Iron: 1mg | Vitamin D: 0% DV

# Whole meal Banana Muffins

**Prep Time:** 15 minutes | **Cooking Time:** 20 minutes | **Total Time:** 35 minutes | **Serving:** 12 | **Cooking Difficulty:** Moderate

**Ingredients:**

- 1 1/2 cups white flour (or a low-fiber flour alternative)
- 1/2 cup sugar
- 1/2 teaspoon baking soda
- 1/2 teaspoon baking powder
- 1/4 teaspoon salt
- 1/2 cup mashed ripe bananas (peeled)
- 1/4 cup vegetable oil
- 1 egg
- 1/4 cup milk (lactose-free if needed)

**Instructions:**

1. Preheat your oven to 350°F (175°C). Line a muffin tin with paper liners.
2. In a bowl, combine the flour, sugar, baking soda, baking powder, and salt.
3. In another bowl, mix the mashed bananas, oil, egg, and milk.
4. Add the wet ingredients to the dry ingredients and stir until just combined.
5. Divide the batter evenly among the muffin cups.
6. Bake for 20 minutes or until a toothpick inserted into the center comes out clean.
7. Let the muffins cool before serving.

**Nutritional Value:** Calories: 180 | Fat: 8g | Saturated Fat: 1g | Cholesterol: 30mg | Sodium: 180mg | Carbohydrate: 24g | Fiber: 1g | Added Sugar: 8g | Protein: 3g | Calcium: 60mg | Potassium: 150mg | Phosphorus: 90mg | Iron: 1mg | Vitamin D: 0% DV

# Chapter 3

# Soups and Stews

## Cream of Chicken Soup

**Prep Time:** 10 minutes | **Cooking Time:** 20 minutes | **Total Time:** 30 minutes | **Serving:** 4 | **Cooking Difficulty:** Easy

**Ingredients:**

- 2 cups low-sodium chicken broth
- 1 cup cooked, shredded chicken breast (skinless)
- 1/2 cup heavy cream or lactose-free cream
- 1 tablespoon all-purpose flour (or a low-fiber alternative)
- 1 tablespoon butter or oil
- Salt and pepper, to taste

**Instructions:**

1. In a saucepan, melt the butter or oil over medium heat. Add the flour and cook for 1-2 minutes, stirring constantly.
2. Slowly whisk in the chicken broth and bring to a simmer.
3. Add the shredded chicken and cook for 5 minutes.
4. Stir in the heavy cream and heat until warmed through.
5. Season with salt and pepper to taste.

**Nutritional Value:** Calories: 250 | Fat: 18g | Saturated Fat: 10g | Cholesterol: 85mg | Sodium: 600mg | Carbohydrate: 8g | Fiber: 0g | Added Sugar: 0g | Protein: 15g | Calcium: 100mg | Potassium: 250mg | Phosphorus: 200mg | Iron: 1mg | Vitamin D: 0% DV

# Chicken Noodle Soup (Without Vegetables)

**Prep Time:** 10 minutes | **Cooking Time:** 15 minutes | **Total Time:** 25 minutes | **Serving:** 4 | **Cooking Difficulty:** Easy

Ingredients:

- 4 cups low-sodium chicken broth
- 1 cup cooked, shredded chicken breast (skinless)
- 1 cup egg noodles (or a low-fiber alternative)
- 1 tablespoon butter or oil
- Salt and pepper, to taste

Instructions:

1. In a large pot, bring the chicken broth to a boil.
2. Add the egg noodles and cook according to package instructions.
3. Stir in the shredded chicken and cook until heated through.
4. Season with salt and pepper to taste.

**Nutritional Value:** Calories: 220 | Fat: 8g | Saturated Fat: 2g | Cholesterol: 60mg | Sodium: 650mg | Carbohydrate: 24g | Fiber: 1g | Added Sugar: 0g | Protein: 14g | Calcium: 50mg | Potassium: 200mg | Phosphorus: 150mg | Iron: 1mg | Vitamin D: 0% DV

# Creamy Tomato Soup

**Prep Time:** 10 minutes | **Cooking Time:** 20 minutes | **Total Time:** 30 minutes | **Serving:** 4 | **Cooking Difficulty:** Easy

**Ingredients:**

- 1 can (15 ounces) tomato puree
- 2 cups low-sodium chicken or vegetable broth
- 1/2 cup heavy cream or lactose-free cream
- 1 tablespoon butter or oil
- 1 tablespoon all-purpose flour (or a low-fiber alternative)
- Salt and pepper, to taste

**Instructions:**

1. In a saucepan, melt the butter or oil over medium heat. Add the flour and cook for 1-2 minutes, stirring constantly.
2. Slowly whisk in the tomato puree and broth. Bring to a simmer.
3. Stir in the heavy cream and heat until warmed through.
4. Season with salt and pepper to taste.

**Nutritional Value:** Calories: 180 | Fat: 12g | Saturated Fat: 7g | Cholesterol: 45mg | Sodium: 700mg | Carbohydrate: 16g | Fiber: 1g | Added Sugar: 0g | Protein: 4g | Calcium: 80mg | Potassium: 300mg | Phosphorus: 150mg | Iron: 1mg | Vitamin D: 0% DV

# Chicken and Dumpling Soup

**Prep Time:** 15 minutes | **Cooking Time:** 25 minutes | **Total Time:** 40 minutes | **Serving:** 4 | **Cooking Difficulty:** Moderate

**Ingredients:**

- 4 cups low-sodium chicken broth
- 1 cup cooked, shredded chicken breast (skinless)
- 1 cup all-purpose flour (or a low-fiber alternative)
- 1/2 teaspoon baking powder
- 1/4 teaspoon salt
- 1/2 cup milk (lactose-free if needed)
- 1 tablespoon butter or oil

**Instructions:**

1. In a pot, bring the chicken broth to a boil. Add the shredded chicken.
2. In a bowl, mix the flour, baking powder, salt, milk, and butter to make dumpling batter.
3. Drop spoonfuls of the batter into the boiling broth. Reduce heat and simmer for 15-20 minutes until dumplings are cooked through.
4. Serve hot.

**Nutritional Value:** Calories: 320 | Fat: 10g | Saturated Fat: 5g | Cholesterol: 75mg | Sodium: 700mg | Carbohydrate: 35g | Fiber: 1g | Added Sugar: 0g | Protein: 20g | Calcium: 120mg | Potassium: 250mg | Phosphorus: 200mg | Iron: 2mg | Vitamin D: 0% DV

# Red Lentil Soup

**Prep Time:** 10 minutes | **Cooking Time:** 20 minutes | **Total Time:** 30 minutes | **Serving:** 4 | **Cooking Difficulty:** Easy

Ingredients:

- 1 cup red lentils, rinsed.
- 4 cups low-sodium chicken or vegetable broth
- 1 tablespoon olive oil
- 1 teaspoon ground cumin
- 1/2 teaspoon turmeric
- Salt and pepper, to taste

Instructions:

1. In a pot, heat olive oil over medium heat. Add the cumin and turmeric.
2. Stir in the lentils and broth. Bring to a boil.
3. Reduce heat and simmer for 20 minutes, or until lentils are tender.
4. Season with salt and pepper to taste.

**Nutritional Value:** Calories: 220 | Fat: 6g | Saturated Fat: 1g | Cholesterol: 0mg | Sodium: 600mg | Carbohydrate: 30g | Fiber: 5g | Added Sugar: 0g | Protein: 12g | Calcium: 60mg | Potassium: 400mg | Phosphorus: 150mg | Iron: 2mg | Vitamin D: 0% DV

# Minestrone Soup

**Prep Time:** 15 minutes | **Cooking Time:** 25 minutes | **Total Time:** 40 minutes | **Serving:** 4 | **Cooking Difficulty:** Moderate

**Ingredients:**

- 4 cups low-sodium chicken or vegetable broth
- 1 cup cooked, shredded chicken breast (skinless)
- 1/2 cup small pasta (such as orzo or ditalini)
- 1 cup peeled and diced potatoes.
- 1/2 cup canned tomatoes (without seeds or skin)
- 1 tablespoon olive oil
- 1 teaspoon dried basil
- Salt and pepper, to taste

**Instructions:**

1. In a pot, heat the olive oil over medium heat. Add the potatoes and cook for 5 minutes.
2. Stir in the broth and bring to a boil.
3. Add the pasta and cook until tender.
4. Stir in the shredded chicken and canned tomatoes. Heat through.
5. Season with basil, salt, and pepper.

**Nutritional Value:** Calories: 250 | Fat: 8g | Saturated Fat: 2g | Cholesterol: 60mg | Sodium: 700mg | Carbohydrate: 30g | Fiber: 2g | Added Sugar: 0g | Protein: 15g | Calcium: 100mg | Potassium: 350mg | Phosphorus: 200mg | Iron: 2mg | Vitamin D: 0% DV

# Chapter 4

# Salads and Light Meals

## Tuna Salad on White Bread

**Prep Time:** 10 minutes | **Cooking Time:** 0 minutes | **Total Time:** 10 minutes | **Serving:** 4 | **Cooking Difficulty:** Easy

**Ingredients:**

- 1 can (5 ounces) tuna in water, drained
- 1/4 cup mayonnaise (or lactose-free alternative)
- 1 tablespoon finely chopped celery (optional, can be omitted for lower fiber)
- 1 tablespoon lemon juice
- Salt and pepper, to taste
- 4 slices white bread

**Instructions:**

1. In a bowl, mix the tuna, mayonnaise, celery (if using), lemon juice, salt, and pepper.
2. Spread the tuna salad evenly onto 2 slices of white bread.
3. Top with the remaining slices of bread, cut in half if desired, and serve.

**Nutritional Value:** Calories: 320 | Fat: 15g | Saturated Fat: 2g | Cholesterol: 45mg | Sodium: 500mg | Carbohydrate: 25g | Fiber: 1g | Added Sugar: 1g | Protein: 22g | Calcium: 30mg | Potassium: 350mg | Phosphorus: 150mg | Iron: 2mg | Vitamin D: 0% DV

# Egg Salad Sandwich

**Prep Time:** 10 minutes | **Cooking Time:** 0 minutes | **Total Time:** 10 minutes | **Serving:** 4 | **Cooking Difficulty:** Easy

**Ingredients:**

- 4 hard-boiled eggs, peeled and chopped.
- 1/4 cup mayonnaise (or lactose-free alternative)
- 1 tablespoon Dijon mustard
- Salt and pepper, to taste
- 4 slices white bread

**Instructions:**

1. In a bowl, combine the chopped eggs, mayonnaise, Dijon mustard, salt, and pepper.
2. Spread the egg salad onto 2 slices of white bread.
3. Top with the remaining slices of bread, cut in half if desired, and serve.

**Nutritional Value:** Calories: 290 | Fat: 18g | Saturated Fat: 4g | Cholesterol: 370mg | Sodium: 450mg | Carbohydrate: 20g | Fiber: 1g | Added Sugar: 1g | Protein: 16g | Calcium: 30mg | Potassium: 250mg | Phosphorus: 150mg | Iron: 2mg | Vitamin D: 10% DV

# Chicken Caesar Salad (Without Croutons)

**Prep Time:** 15 minutes | **Cooking Time:** 10 minutes | **Total Time:** 25 minutes | **Serving:** 4 | **Cooking Difficulty:** Easy

**Ingredients:**

- 2 cups cooked, shredded chicken breast (skinless)
- 4 cups romaine lettuce (chopped)
- 1/4 cup Caesar dressing (lactose-free if needed)
- 2 tablespoons grated Parmesan cheese.
- Salt and pepper, to taste

**Instructions:**

1. In a large bowl, combine the shredded chicken and chopped lettuce.
2. Add the Caesar dressing and toss until well coated.
3. Sprinkle with Parmesan cheese and season with salt and pepper to taste.
4. Serve immediately.

**Nutritional Value:** Calories: 330 | Fat: 22g | Saturated Fat: 5g | Cholesterol: 90mg | Sodium: 600mg | Carbohydrate: 10g | Fiber: 2g | Added Sugar: 1g | Protein: 30g | Calcium: 200mg | Potassium: 400mg | Phosphorus: 250mg | Iron: 1mg | Vitamin D: 5% DV

# Tuna Pasta Salad

*Note: Use a low-fiber pasta alternative.*

**Prep Time:** 10 minutes | **Cooking Time:** 10 minutes | **Total Time:** 20 minutes | **Serving:** 4 | **Cooking Difficulty:** Easy

**Ingredients:**

- 2 cups cooked low-fiber pasta (such as white pasta)
- 1 can (5 ounces) tuna in water, drained
- 1/4 cup mayonnaise (or lactose-free alternative)
- 1 tablespoon lemon juice
- Salt and pepper, to taste

**Instructions:**

1. In a large bowl, combine the cooked pasta and tuna.
2. Mix in the mayonnaise and lemon juice.
3. Season with salt and pepper to taste.
4. Chill before serving if desired.

**Nutritional Value:** Calories: 320 | Fat: 16g | Saturated Fat: 2g | Cholesterol: 45mg | Sodium: 500mg | Carbohydrate: 30g | Fiber: 1g | Added Sugar: 1g | Protein: 20g | Calcium: 30mg | Potassium: 300mg | Phosphorus: 150mg | Iron: 1mg | Vitamin D: 0% DV

# Zesty Zucchini Salad

*Note: Zucchini is typically low in fiber when peeled.*

**Prep Time:** 10 minutes | **Cooking Time:** 0 minutes | **Total Time:** 10 minutes | **Serving:** 4 | **Cooking Difficulty:** Easy

**Ingredients:**

- 2 cups peeled and diced zucchini (cooked if preferred)
- 1/4 cup lemon juice
- 2 tablespoons olive oil
- Salt and pepper, to taste

**Instructions:**

1. In a bowl, combine the diced zucchini, lemon juice, and olive oil.
2. Season with salt and pepper to taste.
3. Toss well and serve immediately.

**Nutritional Value:** Calories: 150 | Fat: 14g | Saturated Fat: 2g | Cholesterol: 0mg | Sodium: 200mg | Carbohydrate: 8g | Fiber: 1g | Added Sugar: 0g | Protein: 2g | Calcium: 30mg | Potassium: 250mg | Phosphorus: 30mg | Iron: 1mg | Vitamin D: 0% DV

# Roasted Vegetables & Halloumi Salad

Note: *Use low-fiber vegetables such as peeled carrots.*

**Prep Time:** 15 minutes | **Cooking Time:** 20 minutes | **Total Time:** 35 minutes | **Serving:** 4 | **Cooking Difficulty:** Moderate

**Ingredients:**

- 1 cup peeled and diced carrots.
- 1 cup peeled and diced potatoes.
- 8 ounces Halloumi cheese, sliced.
- 2 tablespoons olive oil
- 1 teaspoon dried thyme
- Salt and pepper, to taste

**Instructions:**

1. Preheat the oven to 400°F (200°C). Toss the carrots and potatoes with olive oil, thyme, salt, and pepper. Spread on a baking sheet and roast for 20 minutes or until tender.
2. In a pan, grill the Halloumi slices until golden brown on both sides.
3. Combine the roasted vegetables and Halloumi in a bowl.
4. Serve warm.

**Nutritional Value:** Calories: 350 | Fat: 22g | Saturated Fat: 10g | Cholesterol: 50mg | Sodium: 600mg | Carbohydrate: 30g | Fiber: 2g | Added Sugar: 0g | Protein: 18g | Calcium: 400mg | Potassium: 600mg | Phosphorus: 300mg | Iron: 2mg | Vitamin D: 0% DV

# Chapter 5

# Sandwiches and Wraps

## Turkey and Swiss Cheese Sandwich

**Prep Time:** 10 minutes | **Cooking Time:** 0 minutes | **Total Time:** 10 minutes | **Serving:** 2 | **Cooking Difficulty:** Easy

**Ingredients:**

- 4 slices white bread
- 4 slices Swiss cheese
- 4 ounces sliced turkey breast (skinless)
- 1 tablespoon mayonnaise (or lactose-free alternative)
- Salt and pepper, to taste

**Instructions:**

1. Spread mayonnaise on 2 slices of white bread.
2. Layer with sliced turkey breast and Swiss cheese.
3. Top with the remaining slices of bread.
4. Cut in half if desired and serve.

**Nutritional Value:** Calories: 300 | Fat: 12g | Saturated Fat: 5g | Cholesterol: 60mg | Sodium: 700mg | Carbohydrate: 30g | Fiber: 1g | Added Sugar: 2g | Protein: 20g | Calcium: 200mg | Potassium: 300mg | Phosphorus: 200mg | Iron: 2mg | Vitamin D: 0% DV

# Grilled Cheese Sandwich

**Prep Time:** 10 minutes | **Cooking Time:** 5 minutes | **Total Time:** 15 minutes | **Serving:** 2 | **Cooking Difficulty:** Easy

**Ingredients:**

- 4 slices white bread
- 4 slices American cheese (or lactose-free alternative)
- 2 tablespoons butter (for grilling)

**Instructions:**

1. Heat a skillet over medium heat.
2. Butter one side of each bread slice.
3. Place 2 slices of bread, butter side down, in the skillet. Top each with 2 slices of cheese.
4. Cover with the remaining slices of bread, butter side up.
5. Grill until golden brown and cheese is melted, about 2-3 minutes per side.
6. Serve warm.

**Nutritional Value:** Calories: 320 | Fat: 18g | Saturated Fat: 10g | Cholesterol: 60mg | Sodium: 700mg | Carbohydrate: 30g | Fiber: 1g | Added Sugar: 2g | Protein: 14g | Calcium: 400mg | Potassium: 200mg | Phosphorus: 250mg | Iron: 1mg | Vitamin D: 10% DV

# Turkey and Cream Cheese Roll-ups

**Prep Time:** 10 minutes | **Cooking Time:** 0 minutes | **Total Time:** 10 minutes | **Serving:** 4 | **Cooking Difficulty:** Easy

**Ingredients:**

- 8 slices deli turkey breast (skinless)
- 4 ounces cream cheese (or lactose-free alternative)
- 1 tablespoon chopped fresh chives (optional)

**Instructions:**

1. Spread a thin layer of cream cheese on each slice of turkey.
2. Roll up the turkey slices tightly.
3. Slice in half if desired and serve.

**Nutritional Value:** Calories: 200 | Fat: 12g | Saturated Fat: 6g | Cholesterol: 60mg | Sodium: 500mg | Carbohydrate: 2g | Fiber: 0g | Added Sugar: 1g | Protein: 22g | Calcium: 30mg | Potassium: 200mg | Phosphorus: 150mg | Iron: 1mg | Vitamin D: 0% DV

# Grilled Chicken Sandwich

**Prep Time:** 15 minutes | **Cooking Time:** 10 minutes | **Total Time:** 25 minutes | **Serving:** 2 | **Cooking Difficulty:** Easy

Ingredients:

- 2 boneless, skinless chicken breasts
- 4 slices white bread
- 2 tablespoons mayonnaise (or lactose-free alternative)
- Salt and pepper, to taste
- 1 tablespoon olive oil

Instructions:

1. Season the chicken breasts with salt and pepper.
2. Heat olive oil in a skillet over medium heat.
3. Cook chicken breasts for 5-6 minutes per side, until fully cooked.
4. Slice the cooked chicken and place on 2 slices of white bread.
5. Spread mayonnaise on the remaining 2 slices of bread and top the sandwiches.
6. Cut in half if desired and serve.

**Nutritional Value:** Calories: 350 | Fat: 16g | Saturated Fat: 3g | Cholesterol: 90mg | Sodium: 600mg | Carbohydrate: 30g | Fiber: 1g | Added Sugar: 2g | Protein: 25g | Calcium: 30mg | Potassium: 400mg | Phosphorus: 250mg | Iron: 2mg | Vitamin D: 0% DV

# Turkey and Avocado Wrap

*Note: Use a low-fiber wrap or tortilla.*

**Prep Time:** 10 minutes | **Cooking Time:** 0 minutes | **Total Time:** 10 minutes | **Serving:** 2 | **Cooking Difficulty:** Easy

**Ingredients:**

- 2 low-fiber tortillas
- 4 ounces sliced turkey breast (skinless)
- 1/2 avocado, sliced
- 2 tablespoons mayonnaise (or lactose-free alternative)
- Salt and pepper, to taste

**Instructions:**

1. Spread mayonnaise on each tortilla.
2. Layer with sliced turkey and avocado.
3. Season with salt and pepper.
4. Roll up the tortillas tightly and cut in half if desired.

**Nutritional Value:** Calories: 300 | Fat: 15g | Saturated Fat: 3g | Cholesterol: 60mg | Sodium: 600mg | Carbohydrate: 25g | Fiber: 2g | Added Sugar: 2g | Protein: 20g | Calcium: 30mg | Potassium: 300mg | Phosphorus: 200mg | Iron: 1mg | Vitamin D: 0% DV

# Falafel & Pitta Burger

*Note: Use a low-fiber pita.*

**Prep Time:** 15 minutes | **Cooking Time:** 10 minutes | **Total Time:** 25 minutes | **Serving:** 2 | **Cooking Difficulty:** Moderate

**Ingredients:**

- 2 low-fiber pita bread
- 4 cooked falafel patties (store-bought or homemade with minimal fiber)
- 2 tablespoons plain yogurt (or lactose-free alternative)
- 1 tablespoon lemon juice
- Salt and pepper, to taste

**Instructions:**

1. Warm the pita bread according to package instructions.
2. In a bowl, mix yogurt with lemon juice, salt, and pepper.
3. Place the falafel patties inside the pita bread.
4. Top with the yogurt sauce.
5. Serve warm.

**Nutritional Value:** Calories: 350 | Fat: 15g | Saturated Fat: 4g | Cholesterol: 10mg | Sodium: 500mg | Carbohydrate: 35g | Fiber: 4g | Added Sugar: 2g | Protein: 15g | Calcium: 100mg | Potassium: 400mg | Phosphorus: 200mg | Iron: 2mg | Vitamin D: 0% DV

# Chapter 6

# Poultry Dishes

## Simple Chicken Breast with White Rice

**Prep Time:** 10 minutes | **Cooking Time:** 20 minutes | **Total Time:** 30 minutes | **Serving:** 4 | **Cooking Difficulty:** Easy

Ingredients:

- 4 boneless, skinless chicken breasts
- 1 cup white rice
- 2 cups chicken broth (low-sodium)
- 1 tablespoon olive oil
- Salt and pepper, to taste

Instructions:

1. Preheat oven to 375°F (190°C).
2. Season chicken breasts with salt and pepper.
3. Heat olive oil in a skillet over medium heat. Sear chicken breasts for 2-3 minutes per side until browned.
4. Transfer chicken breasts to a baking dish and bake for 15-20 minutes until cooked through.
5. Cook white rice according to package instructions, using chicken broth instead of water for added flavor.
6. Serve chicken breasts over a bed of white rice.

**Nutritional Value:** Calories: 350 | Fat: 8g | Saturated Fat: 2g | Cholesterol: 100mg | Sodium: 500mg | Carbohydrate: 35g | Fiber: 1g | Added Sugar: 0g | Protein: 30g | Calcium: 20mg | Potassium: 400mg | Phosphorus: 300mg | Iron: 2mg | Vitamin D: 0% DV

# Baked Chicken Tenders

**Prep Time:** 15 minutes | **Cooking Time:** 20 minutes | **Total Time:** 35 minutes | **Serving:** 4 | **Cooking Difficulty:** Easy

Ingredients:

- 1 pound chicken tenders
- 1/2 cup all-purpose flour
- 1/2 cup breadcrumbs (low-fiber)
- 1/4 cup grated Parmesan cheese
- 1 egg, beaten
- Salt and pepper, to taste
- Cooking spray

Instructions:

1. Preheat oven to 400°F (200°C).
2. Set up a breading station: place flour in one bowl, beaten egg in another, and a mixture of breadcrumbs and Parmesan in a third.
3. Season chicken tenders with salt and pepper.
4. Dredge chicken tenders in flour, dip in egg, then coat with breadcrumb mixture.
5. Place tenders on a baking sheet sprayed with cooking spray.
6. Bake for 15-20 minutes, turning halfway through, until golden and cooked through.

**Nutritional Value:** Calories: 300 | Fat: 10g | Saturated Fat: 3g | Cholesterol: 100mg | Sodium: 600mg | Carbohydrate: 20g | Fiber: 1g | Added Sugar: 0g | Protein: 25g | Calcium: 200mg | Potassium: 300mg | Phosphorus: 250mg | Iron: 1.5mg | Vitamin D: 0% DV

# Chicken Marsala (Without Mushrooms)

**Prep Time:** 15 minutes | **Cooking Time:** 20 minutes | **Total Time:** 35 minutes | **Serving:** 4 | **Cooking Difficulty:** Moderate

**Ingredients:**

- 4 boneless, skinless chicken breasts
- 1/2 cup all-purpose flour
- 1/2 cup Marsala wine
- 1 cup chicken broth (low-sodium)
- 2 tablespoons olive oil
- 1 tablespoon butter
- Salt and pepper, to taste

**Instructions:**

1. Season chicken breasts with salt and pepper, then dredge in flour.
2. Heat olive oil and butter in a skillet over medium heat.
3. Cook chicken breasts for 5-6 minutes per side until golden brown and cooked through. Remove from skillet and set aside.
4. Deglaze the skillet with Marsala wine, scraping up any browned bits.
5. Add chicken broth and simmer until reduced by half.
6. Return chicken to skillet and coat with sauce. Cook for an additional 2-3 minutes.

**Nutritional Value:** Calories: 300 | Fat: 12g | Saturated Fat: 5g | Cholesterol: 100mg | Sodium: 600mg | Carbohydrate: 10g | Fiber: 1g | Added Sugar: 0g | Protein: 30g | Calcium: 20mg | Potassium: 350mg | Phosphorus: 250mg | Iron: 2mg | Vitamin D: 0% DV

# Chicken Alfredo Pasta

**Prep Time:** 10 minutes | **Cooking Time:** 20 minutes | **Total Time:** 30 minutes | **Serving:** 4 | **Cooking Difficulty:** Moderate

**Ingredients:**

- 2 cups white pasta
- 2 cups cooked, shredded chicken breast
- 1 cup heavy cream
- 1/2 cup grated Parmesan cheese
- 2 tablespoons butter
- Salt and pepper, to taste

**Instructions:**

1. Cook pasta according to package instructions. Drain and set aside.
2. In a skillet, melt butter over medium heat. Add heavy cream and bring to a simmer.
3. Stir in Parmesan cheese and cook until sauce thickens.
4. Add cooked chicken and mix well.
5. Toss with cooked pasta and season with salt and pepper.

**Nutritional Value:** Calories: 450 | Fat: 25g | Saturated Fat: 15g | Cholesterol: 120mg | Sodium: 600mg | Carbohydrate: 35g | Fiber: 1g | Added Sugar: 0g | Protein: 25g | Calcium: 300mg | Potassium: 300mg | Phosphorus: 350mg | Iron: 1.5mg | Vitamin D: 10% DV

# Chicken Teriyaki Bowl

**Prep Time:** 10 minutes | **Cooking Time:** 15 minutes | **Total Time:** 25 minutes | **Serving:** 4 | **Cooking Difficulty:** Easy

Ingredients:

- 1 pound boneless, skinless chicken breast, diced
- 2 cups white rice
- 1/2 cup teriyaki sauce (low-sodium)
- 1 tablespoon olive oil
- Salt and pepper, to taste

Instructions:

1. Cook rice according to package instructions.
2. Heat olive oil in a skillet over medium heat. Add diced chicken and cook until fully cooked.
3. Pour teriyaki sauce over chicken and cook for an additional 2-3 minutes.
4. Serve over a bed of white rice.

**Nutritional Value:** Calories: 350 | Fat: 10g | Saturated Fat: 2g | Cholesterol: 75mg | Sodium: 800mg | Carbohydrate: 40g | Fiber: 1g | Added Sugar: 5g | Protein: 25g | Calcium: 20mg | Potassium: 300mg | Phosphorus: 250mg | Iron: 1.5mg | Vitamin D: 0% DV

# Chicken and Rice Casserole

**Prep Time:** 15 minutes | **Cooking Time:** 40 minutes | **Total Time:** 55 minutes | **Serving:** 4 | **Cooking Difficulty:** Moderate

**Ingredients:**

- 2 cups cooked white rice
- 2 cups cooked, shredded chicken breast
- 1 can cream of chicken soup (low-sodium)
- 1/2 cup milk (lactose-free if needed)
- 1/2 cup grated cheddar cheese
- 1/4 cup melted butter
- Salt and pepper, to taste

**Instructions:**

1. Preheat oven to 350°F (175°C).
2. In a large bowl, combine cooked rice, shredded chicken, cream of chicken soup, milk, cheese, and melted butter. Season with salt and pepper.
3. Transfer mixture to a greased baking dish.
4. Bake for 30-40 minutes, until heated through and bubbly.

**Nutritional Value:** Calories: 400 | Fat: 18g | Saturated Fat: 10g | Cholesterol: 80mg | Sodium: 800mg | Carbohydrate: 40g | Fiber: 1g | Added Sugar: 2g | Protein: 25g | Calcium: 250mg | Potassium: 300mg | Phosphorus: 300mg | Iron: 1.5mg | Vitamin D: 0% DV

# One Pot Chicken and Rice

**Prep Time:** 10 minutes | **Cooking Time:** 30 minutes | **Total Time:** 40 minutes | **Serving:** 4 | **Cooking Difficulty:** Easy

**Ingredients:**

- 1 pound boneless, skinless chicken thighs
- 1 cup white rice
- 2 cups chicken broth (low-sodium)
- 1 tablespoon olive oil
- 1 teaspoon dried thyme
- Salt and pepper, to taste

**Instructions:**

1. Heat olive oil in a large pot over medium heat. Add chicken thighs and cook until browned on both sides.
2. Remove chicken and set aside. In the same pot, add rice and cook for 1-2 minutes.
3. Return chicken to the pot and add chicken broth and thyme. Bring to a boil.
4. Reduce heat, cover, and simmer for 20 minutes or until rice and chicken are cooked through.

**Nutritional Value:** Calories: 350 | Fat: 15g | Saturated Fat: 3g | Cholesterol: 80mg | Sodium: 600mg | Carbohydrate: 35g | Fiber: 1g | Added Sugar: 0g | Protein: 25g | Calcium: 20mg | Potassium: 300mg | Phosphorus: 250mg | Iron: 1.5mg | Vitamin D: 0% DV

# Chicken Curry & Pilaf Rice

**Prep Time:** 15 minutes | **Cooking Time:** 30 minutes | **Total Time:** 45 minutes | **Serving:** 4 | **Cooking Difficulty:** Moderate

**Ingredients:**

- 1 pound boneless, skinless chicken breast, cubed
- 1 cup white rice
- 1 cup chicken broth (low-sodium)
- 1 cup coconut milk
- 2 tablespoons curry powder
- 1 tablespoon olive oil
- Salt and pepper, to taste

**Instructions:**

1. Cook rice according to package instructions.
2. Heat olive oil in a skillet over medium heat. Add cubed chicken and cook until browned and cooked through.
3. Stir in curry powder and cook for 1 minute.
4. Add chicken broth and coconut milk. Simmer for 15 minutes.
5. Serve curry over pilaf rice.

**Nutritional Value:** Calories: 400 | Fat: 20g | Saturated Fat: 12g | Cholesterol: 70mg | Sodium: 600mg | Carbohydrate: 35g | Fiber: 1g | Added Sugar: 2g | Protein: 25g | Calcium: 20mg | Potassium: 400mg | Phosphorus: 300mg | Iron: 1.5mg | Vitamin D: 0% DV

# Chicken and Vegetable Patties

Note: *Use low-fiber vegetables such as zucchini and peeled carrots.*

**Prep Time:** 15 minutes | **Cooking Time:** 20 minutes | **Total Time:** 35 minutes | **Serving:** 4 | **Cooking Difficulty:** Moderate

**Ingredients:**

- 1 pound ground chicken
- 1/2 cup finely grated zucchini (peeled)
- 1/2 cup finely grated peeled carrot
- 1/4 cup breadcrumbs (low-fiber)
- 1 egg
- Salt and pepper, to taste
- 1 tablespoon olive oil

**Instructions:**

1. Preheat oven to 375°F (190°C).
2. In a large bowl, combine ground chicken, grated zucchini, grated carrot, breadcrumbs, egg, salt, and pepper.
3. Form mixture into patties and place on a baking sheet.
4. Brush with olive oil and bake for 15-20 minutes, until cooked through and golden brown.

**Nutritional Value:** Calories: 250 | Fat: 10g | Saturated Fat: 3g | Cholesterol: 80mg | Sodium: 400mg | Carbohydrate: 15g | Fiber: 2g | Added Sugar: 1g | Protein: 25g | Calcium: 30mg | Potassium: 300mg | Phosphorus: 200mg | Iron: 1.5mg | Vitamin D: 0% DV

# Poached Chicken Breast with Rice Pilaf

**Prep Time:** 10 minutes | **Cooking Time:** 20 minutes | **Total Time:** 30 minutes | **Serving:** 4 | **Cooking Difficulty:** Easy

Ingredients:

- 4 boneless, skinless chicken breasts
- 1 cup white rice
- 2 cups chicken broth (low-sodium)
- 1 tablespoon olive oil
- Salt and pepper, to taste

Instructions:

1. Cook white rice according to package instructions using chicken broth for added flavor.
2. In a large pot, add enough water to cover the chicken breasts. Bring to a simmer.
3. Add chicken breasts and cook gently for 15-20 minutes until fully cooked.
4. Remove chicken from the pot and slice. Serve over rice pilaf.

**Nutritional Value:** Calories: 350 | Fat: 8g | Saturated Fat: 2g | Cholesterol: 100mg | Sodium: 500mg | Carbohydrate: 35g | Fiber: 1g | Added Sugar: 0g | Protein: 30g | Calcium: 20mg | Potassium: 400mg | Phosphorus: 300mg | Iron: 2mg | Vitamin D: 0% DV

# Chapter 7

# Beef and Pork Dishes

## Lean Turkey Meatloaf

**Prep Time:** 15 minutes | **Cooking Time:** 50 minutes | **Total Time:** 1 hour 5 minutes | **Serving:** 4 | **Cooking Difficulty:** Moderate

**Ingredients:**

- 1 pound lean ground turkey
- 1/2 cup breadcrumbs (low-fiber)
- 1/4 cup grated Parmesan cheese
- 1/4 cup milk (lactose-free if needed)
- 1 egg
- 2 tablespoons ketchup
- 1 teaspoon dried thyme
- Salt and pepper, to taste

**Instructions:**

1. Preheat oven to 375°F (190°C).
2. In a large bowl, combine ground turkey, breadcrumbs, Parmesan cheese, milk, egg, ketchup, thyme, salt, and pepper.
3. Transfer mixture to a loaf pan and shape into a loaf.
4. Bake for 50 minutes, or until cooked through and internal temperature reaches 165°F (74°C).
5. Let rest for 10 minutes before slicing.

**Nutritional Value:** Calories: 320 | Fat: 14g | Saturated Fat: 4g | Cholesterol: 130mg | Sodium: 600mg | Carbohydrate: 15g | Fiber: 1g | Added Sugar: 2g | Protein: 35g | Calcium: 150mg | Potassium: 400mg | Phosphorus: 300mg | Iron: 2mg | Vitamin D: 0% DV

# Lean Beef Stir-Fry with White Rice

**Prep Time:** 15 minutes | **Cooking Time:** 15 minutes | **Total Time:** 30 minutes | **Serving:** 4 | **Cooking Difficulty:** Easy

**Ingredients:**

- 1 pound lean beef sirloin, thinly sliced
- 2 cups white rice
- 1/2 cup low-sodium soy sauce
- 2 tablespoons vegetable oil
- 1 tablespoon cornstarch
- 1/2 cup water
- Salt and pepper, to taste

**Instructions:**

1. Cook white rice according to package instructions.
2. In a small bowl, mix soy sauce, cornstarch, and water to make a sauce.
3. Heat vegetable oil in a skillet over medium-high heat.
4. Add sliced beef and cook until browned and cooked through, about 5-7 minutes.
5. Pour sauce over beef and cook for an additional 2-3 minutes until thickened.
6. Serve beef stir-fry over white rice.

**Nutritional Value:** Calories: 350 | Fat: 12g | Saturated Fat: 4g | Cholesterol: 80mg | Sodium: 700mg | Carbohydrate: 40g | Fiber: 1g | Added Sugar: 1g | Protein: 25g | Calcium: 20mg | Potassium: 300mg | Phosphorus: 250mg | Iron: 2mg | Vitamin D: 0% DV

# Grilled Pork Chops with Applesauce

**Prep Time:** 10 minutes | **Cooking Time:** 15 minutes | **Total Time:** 25 minutes | **Serving:** 4 | **Cooking Difficulty:** Easy

Ingredients:

- 4 boneless pork chops
- 1 cup applesauce (unsweetened)
- 1 tablespoon olive oil
- Salt and pepper, to taste

Instructions:

1. Preheat grill to medium-high heat.
2. Season pork chops with salt and pepper.
3. Brush with olive oil and grill for 6-8 minutes per side, or until internal temperature reaches 145°F (63°C).
4. Serve with a side of applesauce.

**Nutritional Value:** Calories: 300 | Fat: 15g | Saturated Fat: 4g | Cholesterol: 80mg | Sodium: 400mg | Carbohydrate: 15g | Fiber: 1g | Added Sugar: 0g | Protein: 30g | Calcium: 20mg | Potassium: 350mg | Phosphorus: 250mg | Iron: 2mg | Vitamin D: 0% DV

# Lean Ground Beef Patty with White Rice

**Prep Time:** 10 minutes | **Cooking Time:** 15 minutes | **Total Time:** 25 minutes | **Serving:** 4 | **Cooking Difficulty:** Easy

**Ingredients:**

- 1 pound lean ground beef
- 1 cup white rice
- 1 egg
- 1/2 cup breadcrumbs (low-fiber)
- 1 tablespoon olive oil
- Salt and pepper, to taste

**Instructions:**

1. Cook white rice according to package instructions.
2. In a bowl, mix ground beef with egg, breadcrumbs, salt, and pepper.
3. Shape into 4 patties.
4. Heat olive oil in a skillet over medium heat and cook patties for 5-7 minutes per side, or until cooked through.
5. Serve beef patties over white rice.

**Nutritional Value:** Calories: 350 | Fat: 20g | Saturated Fat: 8g | Cholesterol: 90mg | Sodium: 500mg | Carbohydrate: 30g | Fiber: 1g | Added Sugar: 0g | Protein: 25g | Calcium: 20mg | Potassium: 350mg | Phosphorus: 300mg | Iron: 2mg | Vitamin D: 0% DV

# Baked Pork Loin with Gravy

**Prep Time:** 10 minutes | **Cooking Time:** 50 minutes | **Total Time:** 1 hour | **Serving:** 4 | **Cooking Difficulty:** Moderate

**Ingredients:**

- 1.5 pounds pork loin
- 1 cup low-sodium chicken broth
- 1 tablespoon olive oil
- 1 tablespoon all-purpose flour
- Salt and pepper, to taste

**Instructions:**

1. Preheat oven to 375°F (190°C).
2. Season pork loin with salt and pepper and rub with olive oil.
3. Place pork loin in a roasting pan and bake for 50 minutes, or until internal temperature reaches 145°F (63°C).
4. Remove pork from pan and let rest for 10 minutes.
5. For gravy, heat chicken broth in a pan. Mix flour with a small amount of water and add to broth, whisking until thickened.
6. Slice pork loin and serve with gravy.

**Nutritional Value:** Calories: 350 | Fat: 12g | Saturated Fat: 4g | Cholesterol: 100mg | Sodium: 500mg | Carbohydrate: 10g | Fiber: 1g | Added Sugar: 0g | Protein: 40g | Calcium: 20mg | Potassium: 400mg | Phosphorus: 300mg | Iron: 2mg | Vitamin D: 0% DV

# Lean Beef Stroganoff with Egg Noodles

**Prep Time:** 10 minutes | **Cooking Time:** 20 minutes | **Total Time:** 30 minutes | **Serving:** 4 | **Cooking Difficulty:** Moderate

**Ingredients:**

- 1 pound lean beef sirloin, thinly sliced
- 2 cups egg noodles
- 1 cup low-fat sour cream
- 1 cup beef broth (low-sodium)
- 1 tablespoon olive oil
- 1 tablespoon all-purpose flour
- Salt and pepper, to taste

**Instructions:**

1. Cook egg noodles according to package instructions.
2. Heat olive oil in a skillet over medium heat. Add beef and cook until browned.
3. Stir in flour and cook for 1 minute. Add beef broth and simmer until thickened.
4. Stir in sour cream and season with salt and pepper.
5. Serve beef stroganoff over egg noodles.

**Nutritional Value:** Calories: 400 | Fat: 18g | Saturated Fat: 7g | Cholesterol: 90mg | Sodium: 600mg | Carbohydrate: 35g | Fiber: 2g | Added Sugar: 2g | Protein: 25g | Calcium: 100mg | Potassium: 300mg | Phosphorus: 300mg | Iron: 3mg | Vitamin D: 0% DV

# Lean Meatballs with White Pasta

**Prep Time:** 15 minutes | **Cooking Time:** 20 minutes | **Total Time:** 35 minutes | **Serving:** 4 | **Cooking Difficulty:** Moderate

**Ingredients:**

- 1 pound lean ground beef
- 1/2 cup breadcrumbs (low-fiber)
- 1/4 cup grated Parmesan cheese
- 1 egg
- 2 cups white pasta
- 1 cup marinara sauce (low-fiber)
- Salt and pepper, to taste

**Instructions:**

1. Preheat oven to 375°F (190°C).
2. In a bowl, mix ground beef, breadcrumbs, Parmesan cheese, egg, salt, and pepper.
3. Shape into meatballs and place on a baking sheet.
4. Bake for 20 minutes, or until cooked through.
5. Cook white pasta according to package instructions. Heat marinara sauce in a pan.
6. Serve meatballs over pasta with marinara sauce.

**Nutritional Value:** Calories: 350 | Fat: 18g | Saturated Fat: 6g | Cholesterol: 90mg | Sodium: 700mg | Carbohydrate: 30g | Fiber: 2g | Added Sugar: 3g | Protein: 25g | Calcium: 150mg | Potassium: 350mg | Phosphorus: 300mg | Iron: 3mg | Vitamin D: 0% DV

# Lean Beef Pot Roast (without vegetables)

**Prep Time:** 10 minutes | **Cooking Time:** 3 hours | **Total Time:** 3 hours 10 minutes | **Serving:** 6 | **Cooking Difficulty:** Moderate

Ingredients:

- 3 pounds lean beef chuck roast
- 2 cups low-sodium beef broth
- 1 tablespoon olive oil
- 1 tablespoon all-purpose flour
- Salt and pepper, to taste

Instructions:

1. Preheat oven to 325°F (163°C).
2. Season roast with salt and pepper.
3. Heat olive oil in a large pot over medium-high heat. Brown the roast on all sides.
4. Transfer roast to a roasting pan and pour beef broth over it.
5. Cover and roast for 3 hours, or until tender.
6. Let roast rest before slicing.

**Nutritional Value:** Calories: 400 | Fat: 20g | Saturated Fat: 8g | Cholesterol: 120mg | Sodium: 500mg | Carbohydrate: 10g | Fiber: 0g | Added Sugar: 0g | Protein: 50g | Calcium: 20mg | Potassium: 400mg | Phosphorus: 300mg | Iron: 3mg | Vitamin D: 0% DV

# Lean Beef Lasagna (without ricotta)

**Prep Time:** 20 minutes | **Cooking Time:** 45 minutes | **Total Time:** 1 hour 5 minutes | **Serving:** 6 | **Cooking Difficulty:** Moderate

**Ingredients:**

- 1 pound lean ground beef
- 9 lasagna noodles (low-fiber)
- 2 cups marinara sauce (low-fiber)
- 1 cup shredded mozzarella cheese
- 1 cup grated Parmesan cheese
- 1 egg
- Salt and pepper, to taste

**Instructions:**

1. Preheat oven to 375°F (190°C).
2. Cook lasagna noodles according to package instructions.
3. In a skillet, brown ground beef. Drain excess fat and stir in marinara sauce.
4. In a bowl, mix egg with Parmesan cheese.
5. In a baking dish, layer noodles, beef sauce, and cheese mixture.
6. Top with mozzarella cheese and bake for 45 minutes.

**Nutritional Value:** Calories: 400 | Fat: 20g | Saturated Fat: 8g | Cholesterol: 80mg | Sodium: 600mg | Carbohydrate: 30g | Fiber: 2g | Added Sugar: 4g | Protein: 30g | Calcium: 300mg | Potassium: 350mg | Phosphorus: 300mg | Iron: 3mg | Vitamin D: 0% DV

# Grilled Pork Tenderloin with White Rice

**Prep Time:** 10 minutes | **Cooking Time:** 20 minutes | **Total Time:** 30 minutes | **Serving:** 4 | **Cooking Difficulty:** Easy

Ingredients:

- 1 pound pork tenderloin
- 2 cups white rice
- 1 tablespoon olive oil
- Salt and pepper, to taste

Instructions:

1. Cook white rice according to package instructions.
2. Season pork tenderloin with salt and pepper.
3. Heat olive oil in a grill pan over medium-high heat.
4. Grill pork for 10 minutes per side, or until internal temperature reaches 145°F (63°C).
5. Let rest before slicing. Serve over white rice.

**Nutritional Value:** Calories: 350 | Fat: 10g | Saturated Fat: 3g | Cholesterol: 80mg | Sodium: 400mg | Carbohydrate: 35g | Fiber: 1g | Added Sugar: 0g | Protein: 30g | Calcium: 20mg | Potassium: 350mg | Phosphorus: 250mg | Iron: 2mg | Vitamin D: 0% DV

# Chapter 8

# Seafood Dishes

## Baked Cod with Lemon Butter

**Prep Time:** 10 minutes | **Cooking Time:** 15 minutes | **Total Time:** 25 minutes | **Serving:** 4 | **Cooking Difficulty:** Easy

**Ingredients:**

- 4 cod fillets
- 2 tablespoons unsalted butter, melted
- 1 tablespoon lemon juice
- 1/2 teaspoon dried thyme
- Salt and pepper, to taste

**Instructions:**

1. Preheat oven to 375°F (190°C).
2. Place cod fillets on a baking sheet.
3. In a small bowl, mix melted butter, lemon juice, thyme, salt, and pepper.
4. Brush the mixture over the cod fillets.
5. Bake for 15 minutes, or until the fish flakes easily with a fork.

**Nutritional Value:** Calories: 180 | Fat: 8g | Saturated Fat: 4g | Cholesterol: 60mg | Sodium: 350mg | Carbohydrate: 1g | Fiber: 0g | Added Sugar: 0g | Protein: 25g | Calcium: 30mg | Potassium: 400mg | Phosphorus: 250mg | Iron: 1mg | Vitamin D: 10% DV

# Poached Salmon with Dill Sauce

**Prep Time:** 10 minutes | **Cooking Time:** 15 minutes | **Total Time:** 25 minutes | **Serving:** 4 | **Cooking Difficulty:** Easy

**Ingredients:**

- 4 salmon fillets
- 2 cups water
- 1/2 cup low-sodium chicken broth
- 1 tablespoon lemon juice
- 1 tablespoon fresh dill, chopped
- 1/2 cup sour cream (low-fat)
- Salt and pepper, to taste

**Instructions:**

1. In a large skillet, combine water, chicken broth, and lemon juice. Bring to a simmer.
2. Add salmon fillets, cover, and poach for 12-15 minutes, or until the fish is cooked through.
3. In a small bowl, mix sour cream with dill, salt, and pepper.
4. Serve salmon with dill sauce.

**Nutritional Value:** Calories: 220 | Fat: 10g | Saturated Fat: 2g | Cholesterol: 80mg | Sodium: 300mg | Carbohydrate: 2g | Fiber: 0g | Added Sugar: 0g | Protein: 30g | Calcium: 50mg | Potassium: 400mg | Phosphorus: 300mg | Iron: 1mg | Vitamin D: 20% DV

# Baked Tilapia with Herbs

**Prep Time:** 10 minutes | **Cooking Time:** 20 minutes | **Total Time:** 30 minutes | **Serving:** 4 | **Cooking Difficulty:** Easy

**Ingredients:**

- 4 tilapia fillets
- 2 tablespoons olive oil
- 1 teaspoon dried basil
- 1 teaspoon dried oregano
- Salt and pepper, to taste

**Instructions:**

1. Preheat oven to 375°F (190°C).
2. Place tilapia fillets on a baking sheet.
3. Brush with olive oil and sprinkle with basil, oregano, salt, and pepper.
4. Bake for 20 minutes, or until the fish flakes easily with a fork.

**Nutritional Value:** Calories: 190 | Fat: 9g | Saturated Fat: 1g | Cholesterol: 60mg | Sodium: 250mg | Carbohydrate: 0g | Fiber: 0g | Added Sugar: 0g | Protein: 26g | Calcium: 30mg | Potassium: 400mg | Phosphorus: 250mg | Iron: 1mg | Vitamin D: 10% DV

# Steamed White Fish with Lemon

**Prep Time:** 5 minutes | **Cooking Time:** 10 minutes | **Total Time:** 15 minutes | **Serving:** 4 | **Cooking Difficulty:** Easy

Ingredients:

- 4 white fish fillets (e.g., cod or tilapia)
- 1 lemon, thinly sliced
- 1 tablespoon olive oil
- Salt and pepper, to taste

Instructions:

1. Place fish fillets in a steamer basket.
2. Top with lemon slices and drizzle with olive oil.
3. Steam for 10 minutes, or until fish is cooked through and flakes easily.

**Nutritional Value:** Calories: 180 | Fat: 7g | Saturated Fat: 1g | Cholesterol: 60mg | Sodium: 200mg | Carbohydrate: 1g | Fiber: 0g | Added Sugar: 0g | Protein: 28g | Calcium: 30mg | Potassium: 350mg | Phosphorus: 250mg | Iron: 1mg | Vitamin D: 10% DV

# Tilapia Fish Cakes

**Prep Time:** 15 minutes | **Cooking Time:** 20 minutes | **Total Time:** 35 minutes | **Serving:** 4 | **Cooking Difficulty:** Moderate

**Ingredients:**

- 2 cups cooked tilapia, flaked
- 1/2 cup breadcrumbs (low-fiber)
- 1/4 cup mayonnaise
- 1 egg
- 1 tablespoon fresh parsley, chopped
- Salt and pepper, to taste
- 2 tablespoons olive oil

**Instructions:**

1. In a bowl, combine tilapia, breadcrumbs, mayonnaise, egg, parsley, salt, and pepper.
2. Form mixture into patties.
3. Heat olive oil in a skillet over medium heat.
4. Cook patties for 4-5 minutes per side, or until golden brown and cooked through.

**Nutritional Value:** Calories: 250 | Fat: 15g | Saturated Fat: 3g | Cholesterol: 80mg | Sodium: 350mg | Carbohydrate: 15g | Fiber: 1g | Added Sugar: 1g | Protein: 20g | Calcium: 50mg | Potassium: 300mg | Phosphorus: 250mg | Iron: 1mg | Vitamin D: 10% DV

# Baked Salmon with Dill Cream Sauce

**Prep Time:** 10 minutes | **Cooking Time:** 20 minutes | **Total Time:** 30 minutes | **Serving:** 4 | **Cooking Difficulty:** Moderate

Ingredients:

- 4 salmon fillets
- 1 tablespoon olive oil
- Salt and pepper, to taste
- 1/2 cup sour cream (low-fat)
- 1 tablespoon fresh dill, chopped
- 1 tablespoon lemon juice

Instructions:

1. Preheat oven to 375°F (190°C).
2. Place salmon fillets on a baking sheet and brush with olive oil. Season with salt and pepper.
3. Bake for 20 minutes, or until the fish flakes easily with a fork.
4. In a small bowl, mix sour cream, dill, and lemon juice.
5. Serve salmon with dill cream sauce.

**Nutritional Value:** Calories: 220 | Fat: 12g | Saturated Fat: 3g | Cholesterol: 80mg | Sodium: 300mg | Carbohydrate: 2g | Fiber: 0g | Added Sugar: 0g | Protein: 25g | Calcium: 50mg | Potassium: 400mg | Phosphorus: 250mg | Iron: 1mg | Vitamin D: 20% DV

# Baked Fish Sticks

**Prep Time:** 15 minutes | **Cooking Time:** 15 minutes | **Total Time:** 30 minutes | **Serving:** 4 | **Cooking Difficulty:** Easy

**Ingredients:**

- 1 pound white fish fillets (e.g., cod or tilapia), cut into sticks
- 1/2 cup breadcrumbs (low-fiber)
- 1/4 cup grated Parmesan cheese
- 1/4 cup flour
- 1 egg, beaten
- Salt and pepper, to taste
- Cooking spray

**Instructions:**

1. Preheat oven to 400°F (200°C).
2. Set up a breading station: flour in one bowl, beaten egg in another, and breadcrumbs mixed with Parmesan cheese in a third.
3. Dip fish sticks in flour, then egg, and finally coat with breadcrumb mixture.
4. Place fish sticks on a baking sheet lined with parchment paper and spray with cooking spray.
5. Bake for 15 minutes, or until golden brown and cooked through.

**Nutritional Value:** Calories: 250 | Fat: 10g | Saturated Fat: 2g | Cholesterol: 70mg | Sodium: 400mg | Carbohydrate: 20g | Fiber: 1g | Added Sugar: 0g | Protein: 20g | Calcium: 150mg | Potassium: 300mg | Phosphorus: 250mg | Iron: 2mg | Vitamin D: 10% DV

# Tuna Noodle Casserole

**Prep Time:** 10 minutes | **Cooking Time:** 25 minutes | **Total Time:** 35 minutes | **Serving:** 4 | **Cooking Difficulty:** Moderate

**Ingredients:**

- 1 can (5 ounces) tuna, drained
- 2 cups white pasta
- 1 cup low-fat cream of mushroom soup
- 1/2 cup milk (lactose-free if needed)
- 1/2 cup grated cheddar cheese
- Salt and pepper, to taste

**Instructions:**

1. Preheat oven to 350°F (175°C).
2. Cook white pasta according to package instructions.
3. In a bowl, combine tuna, cooked pasta, cream of mushroom soup, milk, cheese, salt, and pepper.
4. Transfer mixture to a baking dish and bake for 25 minutes, or until bubbly and golden.

**Nutritional Value:** Calories: 350 | Fat: 15g | Saturated Fat: 6g | Cholesterol: 50mg | Sodium: 600mg | Carbohydrate: 35g | Fiber: 1g | Added Sugar: 0g | Protein: 20g | Calcium: 200mg | Potassium: 300mg | Phosphorus: 250mg | Iron: 2mg | Vitamin D: 10% DV

# Chapter 9

# Vegetarian and Vegan Dishes

## Mashed Potato Bowl

**Prep Time:** 10 minutes | **Cooking Time:** 20 minutes | **Total Time:** 30 minutes | **Serving:** 4 | **Cooking Difficulty:** Easy

Ingredients:

- 4 medium potatoes, peeled and diced
- 1/4 cup milk (lactose-free if needed)
- 2 tablespoons unsalted butter
- Salt and pepper, to taste
- 1/4 cup grated cheddar cheese (optional)

Instructions:

1. Boil diced potatoes in a pot of salted water until tender, about 15 minutes.
2. Drain and return potatoes to the pot.
3. Add milk and butter, and mash until smooth.
4. Season with salt and pepper.
5. Stir in cheese, if using, until melted.

**Nutritional Value:** Calories: 180 | Fat: 8g | Saturated Fat: 5g | Cholesterol: 25mg | Sodium: 250mg | Carbohydrate: 25g | Fiber: 2g | Added Sugar: 0g | Protein: 4g | Calcium: 100mg | Potassium: 500mg | Phosphorus: 50mg | Iron: 1mg | Vitamin D: 5% DV

# Vegetarian Lasagna

**Prep Time:** 20 minutes | **Cooking Time:** 45 minutes | **Total Time:** 1 hour 5 minutes | **Serving:** 4 | **Cooking Difficulty:** Moderate

**Ingredients:**

- 9 sheets lasagna noodles (low fiber)
- 2 cups ricotta cheese
- 1 cup grated mozzarella cheese.
- 1/2 cup grated Parmesan cheese.
- 2 cups canned tomato sauce (low fiber)
- 1 egg
- 1 teaspoon dried basil
- Salt and pepper, to taste

**Instructions:**

1. Preheat oven to 375°F (190°C).
2. Cook lasagna noodles according to package instructions.
3. In a bowl, mix ricotta cheese, egg, basil, salt, and pepper.
4. Spread a thin layer of tomato sauce on the bottom of a baking dish.
5. Layer 3 noodles, half of the ricotta mixture, and a third of the mozzarella cheese. Repeat layers.
6. Top with remaining tomato sauce and Parmesan cheese.
7. Bake for 45 minutes, or until bubbly and golden.

**Nutritional Value:** Calories: 350 | Fat: 18g | Saturated Fat: 10g | Cholesterol: 80mg | Sodium: 600mg | Carbohydrate: 35g | Fiber: 3g | Added Sugar: 6g | Protein: 20g | Calcium: 400mg | Potassium: 400mg | Phosphorus: 300mg | Iron: 2mg | Vitamin D: 20% DV

# Vegan Chili Con Carne

**Prep Time:** 15 minutes | **Cooking Time:** 30 minutes | **Total Time:** 45 minutes | **Serving:** 4 | **Cooking Difficulty:** Moderate

Ingredients:

- 1 can (15 ounces) diced tomatoes.
- 1 can (15 ounces) kidney beans, drained and rinsed.
- 1 cup vegetable broth (low fiber)
- 1 tablespoon olive oil
- 1 teaspoon ground cumin
- 1 teaspoon paprika
- Salt and pepper, to taste

Instructions:

1. Heat olive oil in a pot over medium heat.
2. Add tomatoes, beans, vegetable broth, cumin, and paprika.
3. Simmer for 30 minutes, stirring occasionally.
4. Season with salt and pepper.

**Nutritional Value:** Calories: 200 | Fat: 6g | Saturated Fat: 1g | Cholesterol: 0mg | Sodium: 300mg | Carbohydrate: 28g | Fiber: 6g | Added Sugar: 4g | Protein: 10g | Calcium: 80mg | Potassium: 400mg | Phosphorus: 150mg | Iron: 3mg | Vitamin D: 0% DV

# Lentil Nut Roast & Roasted Vegetables

**Prep Time:** 15 minutes | **Cooking Time:** 45 minutes | **Total Time:** 1 hour | **Serving:** 4 | **Cooking Difficulty:** Moderate

Ingredients:

- 1 cup cooked lentils (well-cooked and strained)
- 1/2 cup finely chopped nuts (e.g., cashews)
- 1/2 cup breadcrumbs (low fiber)
- 1/2 cup vegetable broth (low fiber)
- 1 tablespoon olive oil
- 1 teaspoon dried thyme
- Salt and pepper, to taste

Instructions:

1. Preheat oven to 375°F (190°C).
2. In a bowl, mix lentils, nuts, breadcrumbs, vegetable broth, olive oil, thyme, salt, and pepper.
3. Transfer mixture to a loaf pan and bake for 45 minutes.
4. For roasted vegetables, toss low-fiber vegetables (e.g., carrots, potatoes) with olive oil, salt, and pepper. Roast in the oven for 30 minutes.

**Nutritional Value:** Calories: 300 | Fat: 15g | Saturated Fat: 3g | Cholesterol: 0mg | Sodium: 250mg | Carbohydrate: 30g | Fiber: 7g | Added Sugar: 0g | Protein: 15g | Calcium: 50mg | Potassium: 400mg | Phosphorus: 200mg | Iron: 3mg | Vitamin D: 0% DV

# Tofu, Cashew & Egg Fried Rice

**Prep Time:** 15 minutes | **Cooking Time:** 20 minutes | **Total Time:** 35 minutes | **Serving:** 4 | **Cooking Difficulty:** Moderate

Ingredients:

- 1 cup cooked white rice.
- 1/2 cup diced tofu.
- 1/4 cup cashews
- 2 eggs, lightly beaten.
- 2 tablespoons soy sauce (low sodium)
- 1 tablespoon olive oil

Instructions:

1. Heat olive oil in a skillet over medium heat.
2. Add tofu and cook until golden brown. Remove and set aside.
3. In the same skillet, scramble the eggs until cooked through.
4. Add rice, tofu, cashews, and soy sauce. Stir until well combined and heated through.

**Nutritional Value:** Calories: 250 | Fat: 12g | Saturated Fat: 2g | Cholesterol: 180mg | Sodium: 400mg | Carbohydrate: 25g | Fiber: 2g | Added Sugar: 0g | Protein: 14g | Calcium: 50mg | Potassium: 300mg | Phosphorus: 200mg | Iron: 2mg | Vitamin D: 10% DV

# Maple-glazed Tofu Roast

**Prep Time:** 15 minutes | **Cooking Time:** 30 minutes | **Total Time:** 45 minutes | **Serving:** 4 | **Cooking Difficulty:** Moderate

**Ingredients:**

- 1 block (14 ounces) firm tofu pressed and cubed.
- 2 tablespoons maple syrup
- 1 tablespoon soy sauce (low sodium)
- 1 tablespoon olive oil
- 1 teaspoon garlic powder

**Instructions:**

1. Preheat oven to 375°F (190°C).
2. In a bowl, mix maple syrup, soy sauce, olive oil, and garlic powder.
3. Toss tofu cubes in the mixture and spread on a baking sheet.
4. Bake for 30 minutes, stirring halfway through.

**Nutritional Value:** Calories: 180 | Fat: 10g | Saturated Fat: 1g | Cholesterol: 0mg | Sodium: 300mg | Carbohydrate: 16g | Fiber: 2g | Added Sugar: 10g | Protein: 10g | Calcium: 100mg | Potassium: 300mg | Phosphorus: 250mg | Iron: 2mg | Vitamin D: 0% DV

# Penne Pasta

**Prep Time:** 10 minutes | **Cooking Time:** 15 minutes | **Total Time:** 25 minutes | **Serving:** 4 | **Cooking Difficulty:** Easy

**Ingredients:**

- 2 cups penne pasta
- 1 tablespoon olive oil
- Salt, to taste
- Grated Parmesan cheese (optional)

**Instructions:**

1. Cook penne pasta according to package instructions.
2. Drain and toss with olive oil.
3. Season with salt and top with Parmesan cheese if desired.

**Nutritional Value:** Calories: 200 | Fat: 4g | Saturated Fat: 0g | Cholesterol: 0mg | Sodium: 200mg | Carbohydrate: 40g | Fiber: 2g | Added Sugar: 0g | Protein: 7g | Calcium: 30mg | Potassium: 200mg | Phosphorus: 150mg | Iron: 1mg | Vitamin D: 0% DV

# Cheesy Veggie & Herb Muffins

**Prep Time:** 15 minutes | **Cooking Time:** 25 minutes | **Total Time:** 40 minutes | **Serving:** 6 | **Cooking Difficulty:** Moderate

**Ingredients:**

- 1 cup all-purpose flour
- 1/2 cup grated cheddar cheese.
- 1/2 cup finely chopped low-fiber vegetables (e.g., carrots, zucchini, well-cooked)
- 1/4 cup milk (lactose-free if needed)
- 1/4 cup olive oil
- 1 egg
- 1 teaspoon dried herbs (e.g., basil, thyme)
- 1 teaspoon baking powder
- Salt, to taste

**Instructions:**

1. Preheat oven to 375°F (190°C) and line a muffin tin with paper liners.
2. In a bowl, combine flour, baking powder, salt, and herbs.
3. In another bowl, whisk together egg, milk, and olive oil.
4. Add wet ingredients to dry ingredients and mix until just combined. Fold in cheese and chopped vegetables.
5. Divide batter evenly among muffin cups and bake for 25 minutes, or until golden and a toothpick inserted in the center comes out clean.

**Nutritional Value:** Calories: 220 | Fat: 12g | Saturated Fat: 5g | Cholesterol: 55mg | Sodium: 300mg | Carbohydrate: 22g | Fiber: 1g | Added Sugar: 0g | Protein: 8g | Calcium: 150mg | Potassium: 150mg | Phosphorus: 150mg | Iron: 1mg | Vitamin D: 0% DV

# Chapter 10

# Turkey Dishes

## Turkey Burger on a White Bun

**Prep Time:** 10 minutes | **Cooking Time:** 15 minutes | **Total Time:** 25 minutes | **Serving:** 4 | **Cooking Difficulty:** Easy

**Ingredients:**

- 1 pound ground turkey
- 1/4 cup grated Parmesan cheese.
- 1 egg
- 1 tablespoon olive oil
- Salt and pepper, to taste
- 4 white hamburger buns (soft)
- Mayonnaise or mustard, for serving (optional)

**Instructions:**

1. Preheat a grill or skillet over medium heat.
2. In a bowl, combine ground turkey, Parmesan cheese, egg, salt, and pepper. Mix until well combined.
3. Form mixture into 4 patties.
4. Cook patties on the grill or skillet for about 7-8 minutes per side, or until fully cooked and internal temperature reaches 165°F (74°C).
5. Serve on white buns with mayonnaise or mustard if desired.

**Nutritional Value:** Calories: 320 | Fat: 15g | Saturated Fat: 5g | Cholesterol: 95mg | Sodium: 350mg | Carbohydrate: 25g | Fiber: 1g | Added Sugar: 1g | Protein: 25g | Calcium: 150mg | Potassium: 350mg | Phosphorus: 200mg | Iron: 2mg | Vitamin D: 0% DV

# Turkey Tetrazzini

**Prep Time:** 15 minutes | **Cooking Time:** 30 minutes | **Total Time:** 45 minutes | **Serving:** 4 | **Cooking Difficulty:** Moderate

Ingredients:

- 2 cups cooked turkey, diced (without skin)
- 2 cups low-fiber pasta (e.g., white penne or macaroni)
- 1 cup low-sodium chicken broth
- 1 cup heavy cream
- 1/2 cup grated Parmesan cheese
- 1 tablespoon olive oil
- 1 teaspoon dried thyme
- Salt and pepper, to taste

Instructions:

1. Preheat oven to 375°F (190°C).
2. Cook pasta according to package instructions and drain.
3. In a saucepan, heat olive oil over medium heat. Add chicken broth and cream, and bring to a simmer.
4. Stir in Parmesan cheese, thyme, salt, and pepper.
5. Combine cooked turkey and pasta with the sauce and mix well.
6. Transfer mixture to a baking dish and bake for 30 minutes, or until bubbly and golden on top.

**Nutritional Value:** Calories: 450 | Fat: 22g | Saturated Fat: 12g | Cholesterol: 100mg | Sodium: 600mg | Carbohydrate: 38g | Fiber: 2g | Added Sugar: 2g | Protein: 25g | Calcium: 300mg | Potassium: 300mg | Phosphorus: 250mg | Iron: 2mg | Vitamin D: 0% DV

# Turkey Meatballs with Quinoa Pasta

**Prep Time:** 15 minutes | **Cooking Time:** 25 minutes | **Total Time:** 40 minutes | **Serving:** 4 | **Cooking Difficulty:** Moderate

**Ingredients:**

- 1 pound ground turkey
- 1/2 cup breadcrumbs (low-fiber)
- 1/4 cup grated Parmesan cheese
- 1 egg
- 1 tablespoon olive oil
- 1 cup quinoa pasta
- 1 cup low-sodium tomato sauce
- 1 teaspoon dried basil
- Salt and pepper, to taste

**Instructions:**

1. Preheat oven to 375°F (190°C).
2. In a bowl, mix ground turkey, breadcrumbs, Parmesan cheese, egg, salt, and pepper.
3. Form mixture into 16 meatballs and place on a baking sheet.
4. Bake meatballs for 20 minutes, or until fully cooked and internal temperature reaches 165°F (74°C).
5. Meanwhile, cook quinoa pasta according to package instructions and drain.
6. Heat tomato sauce with basil in a saucepan.
7. Combine meatballs with tomato sauce and serve over quinoa pasta.

**Nutritional Value:** Calories: 400 | Fat: 18g | Saturated Fat: 6g | Cholesterol: 120mg | Sodium: 500mg | Carbohydrate: 32g | Fiber: 2g | Added Sugar: 4g | Protein: 25g | Calcium: 150mg | Potassium: 400mg | Phosphorus: 250mg | Iron: 2mg | Vitamin D: 0% DV

# Turkey and Cheese Quesadilla

**Prep Time:** 10 minutes | **Cooking Time:** 10 minutes | **Total Time:** 20 minutes | **Serving:** 2 | **Cooking Difficulty:** Easy

**Ingredients:**

- 2 large flour tortillas (white)
- 1 cup cooked, diced turkey
- 1 cup shredded mild cheddar cheese
- 1 tablespoon olive oil
- Salt and pepper, to taste

**Instructions:**

1. Heat olive oil in a skillet over medium heat.
2. Place one tortilla in the skillet and sprinkle half of the cheese over it.
3. Add turkey on top of the cheese, then sprinkle with the remaining cheese.
4. Top with the second tortilla and cook until golden brown on both sides and cheese is melted.
5. Cut into wedges and serve.

**Nutritional Value:** Calories: 350 | Fat: 18g | Saturated Fat: 8g | Cholesterol: 80mg | Sodium: 500mg | Carbohydrate: 30g | Fiber: 2g | Added Sugar: 0g | Protein: 20g | Calcium: 300mg | Potassium: 200mg | Phosphorus: 250mg | Iron: 1mg | Vitamin D: 0% DV

# Chapter 11

# Baked Goods and Desserts

## Bread and Butter Pudding Festive

**Prep Time:** 20 minutes | **Cooking Time:** 40 minutes | **Total Time:** 1 hour | **Serving:** 6 | **Cooking Difficulty:** Moderate

**Ingredients:**

- 6 slices white bread, crusts removed
- 4 tablespoons unsalted butter
- 2 cups whole milk
- 1/2 cup granulated sugar
- 2 large eggs
- 1 teaspoon vanilla extract
- 1/2 teaspoon ground cinnamon
- 1/4 teaspoon ground nutmeg
- 1/2 cup raisins or currants (optional, if well tolerated)

**Instructions:**

1. Preheat oven to 350°F (175°C).
2. Spread butter on one side of each slice of bread. Cut bread into triangles.
3. Arrange bread slices in a greased baking dish, buttered side up.
4. In a bowl, whisk together milk, sugar, eggs, vanilla extract, cinnamon, and nutmeg.
5. Pour the mixture over the bread slices, pressing down gently to soak.
6. Bake for 35-40 minutes or until the pudding is set and golden brown on top.

**Nutritional Value:** Calories: 250 | Fat: 12g | Saturated Fat: 7g | Cholesterol: 85mg | Sodium: 150mg | Carbohydrate: 30g | Fiber: 1g | Added Sugar: 15g | Protein: 8g | Calcium: 250mg | Potassium: 300mg | Phosphorus: 200mg | Iron: 1mg | Vitamin D: 15% DV

# Broccoli Gratin Festive

**Prep Time:** 15 minutes | **Cooking Time:** 25 minutes | **Total Time:** 40 minutes | **Serving:** 4 | **Cooking Difficulty:** Moderate

**Ingredients:**

- 2 cups broccoli florets (steamed until tender)
- 1 cup shredded cheddar cheese
- 1/2 cup heavy cream
- 1/4 cup grated Parmesan cheese
- 1 tablespoon unsalted butter
- Salt and pepper, to taste

**Instructions:**

1. Preheat oven to 375°F (190°C).
2. Arrange steamed broccoli in a greased baking dish.
3. In a saucepan, melt butter over medium heat. Add heavy cream and bring to a simmer.
4. Stir in cheddar cheese until melted and smooth. Season with salt and pepper.
5. Pour cheese sauce over broccoli and sprinkle with Parmesan cheese.
6. Bake for 20-25 minutes or until the top is golden and bubbly.

**Nutritional Value:** Calories: 320 | Fat: 25g | Saturated Fat: 14g | Cholesterol: 90mg | Sodium: 400mg | Carbohydrate: 6g | Fiber: 2g | Added Sugar: 0g | Protein: 20g | Calcium: 500mg | Potassium: 350mg | Phosphorus: 350mg | Iron: 1mg | Vitamin D: 10% DV

# Vanilla Panna Cotta Berry Compote

**Prep Time:** 10 minutes | **Cooking Time:** 10 minutes | **Total Time:** 3 hours | **Serving:** 4 | **Cooking Difficulty:** Easy

**Ingredients:**

*For the Panna Cotta:*

- 2 cups heavy cream
- 1/2 cup granulated sugar
- 1 teaspoon vanilla extract
- 1 packet (2 1/4 teaspoons) unflavored gelatin

*For the Berry Compote:*

- 1 cup canned or thawed berries (e.g., strawberries or blueberries, well-drained)
- 1/4 cup granulated sugar
- 1 tablespoon lemon juice

**Instructions:**

1. For the panna cotta, heat cream and sugar in a saucepan over medium heat until sugar is dissolved. Do not boil.
2. In a small bowl, dissolve gelatin in 3 tablespoons of warm water. Add to cream mixture and stir until completely dissolved. Remove from heat and stir in vanilla extract.
3. Pour mixture into serving glasses or molds. Chill in the refrigerator for at least 3 hours or until set.
4. For the compote, combine berries, sugar, and lemon juice in a saucepan. Cook over medium heat until sugar is dissolved and berries are softened.
5. Spoon compote over panna cotta before serving.

**Nutritional Value:** Calories: 320 | Fat: 25g | Saturated Fat: 15g | Cholesterol: 85mg | Sodium: 70mg | Carbohydrate: 25g | Fiber: 1g | Added Sugar: 15g | Protein: 4g | Calcium: 150mg | Potassium: 250mg | Phosphorus: 150mg | Iron: 0.5mg | Vitamin D: 10% DV

# Strawberry Cheesecake

**Prep Time:** 15 minutes | **Cooking Time:** 45 minutes | **Total Time:** 2 hours | **Serving:** 8 | **Cooking Difficulty:** Moderate

**Ingredients:**

*For the Crust:*

- 1 1/2 cups graham cracker crumbs
- 1/4 cup granulated sugar
- 6 tablespoons unsalted butter, melted

*For the Filling:*

- 2 (8-ounce) packages cream cheese, softened
- 1 cup granulated sugar
- 2 large eggs
- 1 teaspoon vanilla extract
- 1/2 cup sour cream

*For the Topping:*

- 1 cup strawberry puree (strained)

**Instructions:**

1. Preheat oven to 325°F (163°C). Grease a 9-inch springform pan.
2. Mix graham cracker crumbs, sugar, and melted butter. Press mixture into the bottom of the prepared pan.
3. For the filling, beat cream cheese and sugar until smooth. Add eggs one at a time, beating well after each addition. Stir in vanilla and sour cream.
4. Pour filling over crust and bake for 45 minutes or until set. Turn off the oven and let cheesecake cool in the oven with the door ajar.
5. Refrigerate for at least 4 hours. Top with strawberry puree before serving.

**Nutritional Value:** Calories: 380 | Fat: 28g | Saturated Fat: 16g | Cholesterol: 110mg | Sodium: 300mg | Carbohydrate: 30g | Fiber: 1g | Added Sugar: 20g | Protein: 7g | Calcium: 250mg | Potassium: 200mg | Phosphorus: 200mg | Iron: 1mg | Vitamin D: 5% DV

# Banana Cake

**Prep Time:** 15 minutes | **Cooking Time:** 30 minutes | **Total Time:** 45 minutes | **Serving:** 8 | **Cooking Difficulty:** Moderate

**Ingredients:**

- 1 1/2 cups all-purpose flour
- 1 cup granulated sugar
- 1/2 teaspoon baking powder
- 1/2 teaspoon baking soda
- 1/4 teaspoon salt
- 1/2 cup unsalted butter, softened
- 2 large eggs
- 1 cup mashed ripe bananas (about 2 medium bananas)
- 1/4 cup milk

**Instructions:**

1. Preheat oven to 350°F (175°C). Grease and flour an 8-inch round cake pan.
2. In a bowl, whisk together flour, sugar, baking powder, baking soda, and salt.
3. In a separate bowl, beat butter until creamy. Add eggs one at a time, mixing well after each addition.
4. Stir in mashed bananas and milk until combined.
5. Pour batter into prepared pan and bake for 30-35 minutes or until a toothpick inserted in the center comes out clean.

**Nutritional Value:** Calories: 290 | Fat: 12g | Saturated Fat: 7g | Cholesterol: 55mg | Sodium: 200mg | Carbohydrate: 42g | Fiber: 1g | Added Sugar: 15g | Protein: 4g | Calcium: 60mg | Potassium: 250mg | Phosphorus: 100mg | Iron: 1mg | Vitamin D: 0% DV

# Marbled Brownies

**Prep Time:** 15 minutes | **Cooking Time:** 30 minutes | **Total Time:** 45 minutes | **Serving:** 9 | **Cooking Difficulty:** Moderate

Ingredients:

- 1/2 cup unsalted butter
- 1 cup granulated sugar
- 2 large eggs
- 1 teaspoon vanilla extract
- 1/2 cup all-purpose flour
- 1/4 cup cocoa powder
- 1/4 teaspoon baking powder
- 1/4 teaspoon salt
- 1/2 cup cream cheese, softened
- 1/4 cup granulated sugar (for marbling)

Instructions:

1. Preheat oven to 350°F (175°C). Grease and line an 8-inch square baking pan.
2. Melt butter and mix with sugar, eggs, and vanilla. Stir in flour, cocoa powder, baking powder, and salt until combined.
3. Spread half of the brownie batter into the prepared pan.
4. In a bowl, mix cream cheese with sugar until smooth. Drop spoonfuls of the mixture over the batter and swirl with a knife.
5. Bake for 30 minutes or until set. Let cool before cutting into squares.

**Nutritional Value:** Calories: 280 | Fat: 17g | Saturated Fat: 10g | Cholesterol: 75mg | Sodium: 130mg | Carbohydrate: 30g | Fiber: 1g | Added Sugar: 20g | Protein: 4g | Calcium: 70mg | Potassium: 200mg | Phosphorus: 150mg | Iron: 1mg | Vitamin D: 0% DV

# French Chocolate Pie

**Prep Time:** 15 minutes | **Cooking Time:** 25 minutes | **Total Time:** 1 hour | **Serving:** 8 | **Cooking Difficulty:** Moderate

**Ingredients:**

- 1 pre-made graham cracker pie crust
- 1 cup heavy cream
- 1 cup semi-sweet chocolate chips
- 1/4 cup granulated sugar
- 2 large eggs
- 1 teaspoon vanilla extract

**Instructions:**

1. Preheat oven to 350°F (175°C).
2. Heat heavy cream in a saucepan until just simmering. Remove from heat and stir in chocolate chips until melted and smooth.
3. In a bowl, whisk together sugar, eggs, and vanilla. Stir in chocolate mixture until combined.
4. Pour filling into the pie crust and bake for 20-25 minutes, or until set.
5. Cool completely before slicing.

**Nutritional Value:** Calories: 400 | Fat: 30g | Saturated Fat: 18g | Cholesterol: 110mg | Sodium: 200mg | Carbohydrate: 35g | Fiber: 2g | Added Sugar: 20g | Protein: 5g | Calcium: 80mg | Potassium: 250mg | Phosphorus: 200mg | Iron: 2mg | Vitamin D: 0% DV

# Carrot Cake

**Prep Time:** 20 minutes | **Cooking Time:** 35 minutes | **Total Time:** 1 hour | **Serving:** 8 | **Cooking Difficulty:** Moderate

**Ingredients:**

- 1 1/2 cups all-purpose flour
- 1 cup granulated sugar
- 1/2 teaspoon baking powder
- 1/2 teaspoon baking soda
- 1/4 teaspoon salt
- 1/2 teaspoon ground cinnamon
- 1/2 teaspoon ground nutmeg
- 1/2 cup vegetable oil
- 2 large eggs
- 1 cup finely grated carrots

**Instructions:**

1. Preheat oven to 350°F (175°C). Grease and flour an 8-inch round cake pan.
2. In a bowl, whisk together flour, sugar, baking powder, baking soda, salt, cinnamon, and nutmeg.
3. In another bowl, beat oil and eggs until well combined. Stir in grated carrots.
4. Add dry ingredients to the wet mixture and mix until just combined.
5. Pour batter into prepared pan and bake for 30-35 minutes, or until a toothpick inserted in the center comes out clean.

**Nutritional Value:** Calories: 320 | Fat: 18g | Saturated Fat: 7g | Cholesterol: 50mg | Sodium: 200mg | Carbohydrate: 38g | Fiber: 1g | Added Sugar: 15g | Protein: 4g | Calcium: 60mg | Potassium: 300mg | Phosphorus: 150mg | Iron: 1mg | Vitamin D: 0% DV

# Cream Cheese Frosting

**Prep Time:** 10 minutes | **Cooking Time:** 0 minutes | **Total Time:** 10 minutes | **Serving:** 12 | **Cooking Difficulty:** Easy

**Ingredients:**

- 1 (8-ounce) package cream cheese, softened
- 1/2 cup unsalted butter, softened
- 2 cups powdered sugar
- 1 teaspoon vanilla extract

**Instructions:**

1. In a bowl, beat cream cheese and butter until creamy and smooth.
2. Gradually add powdered sugar, beating well after each addition.
3. Stir in vanilla extract until well combined.
4. Spread or pipe frosting on cooled cakes or cupcakes.

**Nutritional Value:** Calories: 130 | Fat: 10g | Saturated Fat: 6g | Cholesterol: 35mg | Sodium: 75mg | Carbohydrate: 10g | Fiber: 0g | Added Sugar: 9g | Protein: 2g | Calcium: 40mg | Potassium: 60mg | Phosphorus: 50mg | Iron: 0.1mg | Vitamin D: 0% DV

# Chapter 12

# Smoothies and Beverages

## Creamy Banana Vanilla Shake

**Prep Time:** 5 minutes | **Cooking Time:** 0 minutes | **Total Time:** 5 minutes | **Serving:** 2 | **Cooking Difficulty:** Easy

Ingredients:

- 1 ripe banana, peeled
- 1 cup vanilla yogurt (plain, low-fat)
- 1/2 cup milk (whole or 2%)
- 1 teaspoon vanilla extract
- 1/2 cup ice cubes (optional)

Instructions:

1. In a blender, combine banana, vanilla yogurt, milk, and vanilla extract.
2. Blend until smooth. Add ice cubes if desired and blend again.
3. Pour into glasses and serve immediately.

**Nutritional Value:** Calories: 210 | Fat: 4g | Saturated Fat: 2g | Cholesterol: 20mg | Sodium: 90mg | Carbohydrate: 35g | Fiber: 1g | Added Sugar: 15g | Protein: 7g | Calcium: 300mg | Potassium: 400mg | Phosphorus: 250mg | Iron: 0.5mg | Vitamin D: 20% DV

# Smooth Peach Nectar

**Prep Time:** 5 minutes | **Cooking Time:** 0 minutes | **Total Time:** 5 minutes | **Serving:** 2 | **Cooking Difficulty:** Easy

**Ingredients:**

- 1 cup canned peach slices (in juice, well-drained)
- 1 cup water
- 1 tablespoon honey (optional)
- 1/2 teaspoon lemon juice

**Instructions:**

1. In a blender, combine peach slices, water, honey (if using), and lemon juice.
2. Blend until smooth.
3. Pour into glasses and serve chilled.

**Nutritional Value:** Calories: 80 | Fat: 0g | Saturated Fat: 0g | Cholesterol: 0mg | Sodium: 10mg | Carbohydrate: 20g | Fiber: 1g | Added Sugar: 5g | Protein: 0g | Calcium: 15mg | Potassium: 180mg | Phosphorus: 15mg | Iron: 0.2mg | Vitamin D: 0% DV

# Mellow Mango Lassi

**Prep Time:** 5 minutes | **Cooking Time:** 0 minutes | **Total Time:** 5 minutes | **Serving:** 2 | **Cooking Difficulty:** Easy

Ingredients:

- 1 cup plain yogurt (low-fat)
- 1/2 cup mango puree (canned or fresh)
- 1/2 cup water
- 1/2 teaspoon ground cardamom (optional)
- 1 teaspoon honey (optional)

Instructions:

1. In a blender, combine yogurt, mango puree, water, cardamom (if using), and honey (if using).
2. Blend until smooth.
3. Pour into glasses and serve immediately.

**Nutritional Value:** Calories: 150 | Fat: 2g | Saturated Fat: 1g | Cholesterol: 10mg | Sodium: 80mg | Carbohydrate: 30g | Fiber: 1g | Added Sugar: 10g | Protein: 6g | Calcium: 250mg | Potassium: 250mg | Phosphorus: 200mg | Iron: 0.2mg | Vitamin D: 10% DV

# Black Forest Smoothie

**Prep Time:** 5 minutes | **Cooking Time:** 0 minutes | **Total Time:** 5 minutes | **Serving:** 2 | **Cooking Difficulty:** Easy

Ingredients:

- 1 cup canned cherries (in juice, well-drained)
- 1/2 cup vanilla yogurt (plain, low-fat)
- 1/2 cup milk (whole or 2%)
- 1 tablespoon cocoa powder
- 1/2 cup ice cubes (optional)

Instructions:

1. In a blender, combine cherries, vanilla yogurt, milk, and cocoa powder.
2. Blend until smooth. Add ice cubes if desired and blend again.
3. Pour into glasses and serve immediately.

**Nutritional Value:** Calories: 180 | Fat: 3g | Saturated Fat: 2g | Cholesterol: 15mg | Sodium: 90mg | Carbohydrate: 30g | Fiber: 1g | Added Sugar: 12g | Protein: 6g | Calcium: 300mg | Potassium: 250mg | Phosphorus: 200mg | Iron: 0.8mg | Vitamin D: 20% DV

# Silky Strawberry Yogurt Blend

**Prep Time:** 5 minutes | **Cooking Time:** 0 minutes | **Total Time:** 5 minutes | **Serving:** 2 | **Cooking Difficulty:** Easy

**Ingredients:**

- 1 cup plain yogurt (low-fat)
- 1/2 cup strawberry puree (canned or fresh)
- 1/2 cup milk (whole or 2%)
- 1 tablespoon honey (optional)
- 1/2 cup ice cubes (optional)

**Instructions:**

1. In a blender, combine yogurt, strawberry puree, milk, and honey (if using).
2. Blend until smooth. Add ice cubes if desired and blend again.
3. Pour into glasses and serve immediately.

**Nutritional Value:** Calories: 160 | Fat: 2g | Saturated Fat: 1g | Cholesterol: 10mg | Sodium: 80mg | Carbohydrate: 30g | Fiber: 1g | Added Sugar: 12g | Protein: 6g | Calcium: 250mg | Potassium: 200mg | Phosphorus: 200mg | Iron: 0.2mg | Vitamin D: 10% DV

# Chilled Honeydew Mint Refresher

**Prep Time:** 5 minutes | **Cooking Time:** 0 minutes | **Total Time:** 5 minutes | **Serving:** 2 | **Cooking Difficulty:** Easy

**Ingredients:**

- 1 cup honeydew melon, peeled and cubed
- 1/2 cup water
- 1 tablespoon honey (optional)
- 1 tablespoon fresh mint leaves, chopped

**Instructions:**

1. In a blender, combine honeydew melon, water, and honey (if using).
2. Blend until smooth.
3. Stir in chopped mint leaves and serve chilled.

**Nutritional Value:** Calories: 70 | Fat: 0g | Saturated Fat: 0g | Cholesterol: 0mg | Sodium: 10mg | Carbohydrate: 18g | Fiber: 0g | Added Sugar: 5g | Protein: 1g | Calcium: 15mg | Potassium: 250mg | Phosphorus: 10mg | Iron: 0.1mg | Vitamin D: 0% DV

# Velvety Chocolate Almond Milk

**Prep Time:** 5 minutes | **Cooking Time:** 0 minutes | **Total Time:** 5 minutes | **Serving:** 2 | **Cooking Difficulty:** Easy

Ingredients:

- 1 cup almond milk (unsweetened)
- 2 tablespoons cocoa powder
- 1 tablespoon honey or maple syrup
- 1/2 teaspoon vanilla extract

Instructions:

1. In a small bowl, mix cocoa powder with a bit of almond milk to form a paste.
2. In a blender, combine the cocoa paste, remaining almond milk, honey, and vanilla extract.
3. Blend until smooth.
4. Serve chilled or warmed.

**Nutritional Value:** Calories: 80 | Fat: 3g | Saturated Fat: 0g | Cholesterol: 0mg | Sodium: 80mg | Carbohydrate: 10g | Fiber: 1g | Added Sugar: 8g | Protein: 1g | Calcium: 450mg | Potassium: 200mg | Phosphorus: 150mg | Iron: 1mg | Vitamin D: 25% DV

# Tropical Coconut Pineapple Cooler

**Prep Time:** 5 minutes | **Cooking Time:** 0 minutes | **Total Time:** 5 minutes | **Serving:** 2 | **Cooking Difficulty:** Easy

Ingredients:

- 1 cup coconut milk
- 1/2 cup pineapple juice (strained)
- 1 tablespoon honey (optional)
- 1/2 cup ice cubes (optional)

Instructions:

1. In a blender, combine coconut milk, pineapple juice, and honey (if using).
2. Blend until well combined. Add ice cubes if desired and blend again.
3. Pour into glasses and serve immediately.

**Nutritional Value:** Calories: 110 | Fat: 9g | Saturated Fat: 8g | Cholesterol: 0mg | Sodium: 10mg | Carbohydrate: 9g | Fiber: 0g | Added Sugar: 7g | Protein: 1g | Calcium: 50mg | Potassium: 150mg | Phosphorus: 80mg | Iron: 0.2mg | Vitamin D: 10% DV

# Soothing Chamomile Lemon Tea

**Prep Time:** 5 minutes | **Cooking Time:** 5 minutes | **Total Time:** 10 minutes | **Serving:** 2 | **Cooking Difficulty:** Easy

**Ingredients:**

- 2 chamomile tea bags
- 2 cups water
- 1 tablespoon lemon juice
- 1 teaspoon honey (optional)

**Instructions:**

1. Boil water and pour over chamomile tea bags in a teapot or heatproof container.
2. Steep for 5 minutes, then remove tea bags.
3. Stir in lemon juice and honey (if using).
4. Serve warm or chilled.

**Nutritional Value:** Calories: 20 | Fat: 0g | Saturated Fat: 0g | Cholesterol: 0mg | Sodium: 5mg | Carbohydrate: 5g | Fiber: 0g | Added Sugar: 4g | Protein: 0g | Calcium: 10mg | Potassium: 30mg | Phosphorus: 5mg | Iron: 0.1mg | Vitamin D: 0% DV

# Gentle Ginger Pear Sipper

**Prep Time:** 5 minutes | **Cooking Time:** 0 minutes | **Total Time:** 5 minutes | **Serving:** 2 | **Cooking Difficulty:** Easy

**Ingredients:**

- 1 cup pear juice (strained)
- 1/2 cup ginger ale (uncolored)
- 1 tablespoon honey (optional)

**Instructions:**

1. In a blender or pitcher, combine pear juice, ginger ale, and honey (if using).
2. Stir or blend until well combined.
3. Serve chilled.

**Nutritional Value:** Calories: 100 | Fat: 0g | Saturated Fat: 0g | Cholesterol: 0mg | Sodium: 10mg | Carbohydrate: 26g | Fiber: 0g | Added Sugar: 8g | Protein: 0g | Calcium: 0mg | Potassium: 150mg | Phosphorus: 10mg | Iron: 0.2mg | Vitamin D: 0% DV

# Creamy Cantaloupe Cooler

**Prep Time:** 5 minutes | **Cooking Time:** 0 minutes | **Total Time:** 5 minutes | **Serving:** 2 | **Cooking Difficulty:** Easy

Ingredients:

- 1 cup cantaloupe, peeled and cubed
- 1/2 cup plain yogurt (low-fat)
- 1/2 cup water
- 1 tablespoon honey (optional)

Instructions:

1. In a blender, combine cantaloupe, yogurt, water, and honey (if using).
2. Blend until smooth.
3. Pour into glasses and serve immediately.

**Nutritional Value:** Calories: 120 | Fat: 1g | Saturated Fat: 0g | Cholesterol: 5mg | Sodium: 30mg | Carbohydrate: 28g | Fiber: 1g | Added Sugar: 6g | Protein: 3g | Calcium: 150mg | Potassium: 250mg | Phosphorus: 100mg | Iron: 0.3mg | Vitamin D: 5% DV

# Chapter 13

# Meal Plan

| Day | Breakfast | Lunch | Dinner | Snack |
|---|---|---|---|---|
| 1 | Scrambled Eggs with Toast (32) | Tuna Salad on White Bread (44) | Simple Chicken Breast with White Rice (56) | Creamy Banana Vanilla Shake (106) |
| 2 | Egg White Omelet (33) | Egg Salad Sandwich (45) | Baked Chicken Tenders (57) | Smooth Peach Nectar (107) |
| 3 | Poached Eggs on Toast (34) | Chicken Caesar Salad (without croutons) (46) | Chicken Marsala (without mushrooms) (58) | Mellow Mango Lassi (108) |
| 4 | Scrambled Egg Whites with Cheese (35) | Tuna Pasta Salad (47) | Chicken Alfredo Pasta (59) | Black Forest Smoothie (109) |
| 5 | Wholemeal Banana Muffins (36) | Zesty Zucchini Salad (48) | Chicken Teriyaki Bowl (60) | Silky Strawberry Yogurt Blend (110) |

| | | | | |
|---|---|---|---|---|
| 6 | Scrambled Eggs with Toast (32) | Roasted Vegetables & Halloumi Salad (49) | Chicken and Rice Casserole (61) | Chilled Honeydew Mint Refresher (111) |
| 7 | Egg White Omelet (33) | Turkey and Swiss Cheese Sandwich (50) | One Pot Chicken and Rice (62) | Velvety Chocolate Almond Milk (112) |
| 8 | Poached Eggs on Toast (34) | Grilled Cheese Sandwich (51) | Chicken Curry & Pilaf Rice (63) | Tropical Coconut Pineapple Cooler (113) |
| 9 | Scrambled Egg Whites with Cheese (35) | Turkey and Cream Cheese Roll-ups (52) | Chicken and Vegetable Patties (64) | Soothing Chamomile Lemon Tea (114) |
| 10 | Wholemeal Banana Muffins (36) | Grilled Chicken Sandwich (53) | Poached Chicken Breast with Rice Pilaf (65) | Gentle Ginger Pear Sipper (115) |
| 11 | Scrambled Eggs with Toast (32) | Turkey and Avocado Wrap (54) | Baked Cod with Lemon Butter (76) | Creamy Cantaloupe Cooler (116) |
| 12 | Egg White Omelet (33) | Chicken Noodle Soup (without vegetables) (39) | Poached Salmon with Dill Sauce (77) | Creamy Banana Vanilla Shake (106) |

| | | | | |
|---|---|---|---|---|
| 13 | Poached Eggs on Toast (34) | Cream of Chicken Soup (38) | Baked Tilapia with Herbs (78) | Smooth Peach Nectar (107) |
| 14 | Scrambled Egg Whites with Cheese (35) | Creamy Tomato Soup (40) | Steamed White Fish with Lemon (79) | Mellow Mango Lassi (108) |
| 15 | Wholemeal Banana Muffins (36) | Chicken and Dumpling Soup (41) | Tilapia Fish Cakes (80) | Black Forest Smoothie (109) |
| 16 | Scrambled Eggs with Toast (32) | Egg Salad Sandwich (45) | Baked Salmon with Dill Cream Sauce (81) | Silky Strawberry Yogurt Blend (110) |
| 17 | Egg White Omelet (33) | Chicken Caesar Salad (without croutons) (46) | Baked Fish Sticks (82) | Chilled Honeydew Mint Refresher (111) |
| 18 | Poached Eggs on Toast (34) | Tuna Salad on White Bread (44) | Tuna Noodle Casserole (83) | Velvety Chocolate Almond Milk (112) |
| 19 | Scrambled Egg Whites with Cheese (35) | Chicken and Dumpling Soup (41) | Chicken Alfredo Pasta (59) | Tropical Coconut Pineapple Cooler (113) |

| | | | | |
|---|---|---|---|---|
| 20 | Wholemeal Banana Muffins (36) | Zesty Zucchini Salad (48) | Chicken Teriyaki Bowl (60) | Soothing Chamomile Lemon Tea (114) |
| 21 | Scrambled Eggs with Toast (32) | Roasted Vegetables & Halloumi Salad (49) | Chicken and Rice Casserole (61) | Gentle Ginger Pear Sipper (115) |
| 22 | Egg White Omelet (33) | Turkey and Swiss Cheese Sandwich (50) | Poached Chicken Breast with Rice Pilaf (65) | Creamy Cantaloupe Cooler (116) |
| 23 | Poached Eggs on Toast (34) | Grilled Cheese Sandwich (51) | Baked Cod with Lemon Butter (76) | Creamy Banana Vanilla Shake (106) |
| 24 | Scrambled Egg Whites with Cheese (35) | Turkey and Cream Cheese Roll-ups (52) | Baked Tilapia with Herbs (78) | Smooth Peach Nectar (107) |
| 25 | Wholemeal Banana Muffins (36) | Turkey and Avocado Wrap (54) | Steamed White Fish with Lemon (79) | Mellow Mango Lassi (108) |
| 26 | Scrambled Eggs with Toast (32) | Chicken Noodle Soup (without vegetables) (39) | Tilapia Fish Cakes (80) | Black Forest Smoothie (109) |

| | | | | |
|---|---|---|---|---|
| 27 | Egg White Omelet (33) | Cream of Chicken Soup (38) | Baked Salmon with Dill Cream Sauce (81) | Silky Strawberry Yogurt Blend (110) |
| 28 | Poached Eggs on Toast (34) | Egg Salad Sandwich (45) | Chicken Curry & Pilaf Rice (63) | Chilled Honeydew Mint Refresher (111) |
| 29 | Scrambled Egg Whites with Cheese (35) | Tuna Pasta Salad (47) | Chicken and Vegetable Patties (64) | Velvety Chocolate Almond Milk (112) |
| 30 | Wholemeal Banana Muffins (36) | Grilled Chicken Sandwich (53) | Chicken Teriyaki Bowl (60) | Tropical Coconut Pineapple Cooler (113) |

# Chapter 14

# Managing Common Challenges with Diet

## *Tips for Managing Gas, Odor, and Stool Consistency*

Living with a colostomy or ileostomy often requires adjusting to new aspects of digestive health, including managing gas, odor, and stool consistency. While these concerns can be challenging, understanding how to manage them effectively can greatly enhance your comfort and confidence. Here are some practical tips to help you navigate these issues:

**Managing Gas**

1. **Identify and Avoid Gas-Producing Foods:**
   - Certain foods are known to produce more gas, such as beans, carbonated beverages, and cruciferous vegetables like broccoli and cabbage. Keep a food diary to identify any specific triggers and avoid them when possible.

2. **Eat Smaller, Frequent Meals:**
   - Large meals can lead to more gas production. Opt for smaller, more frequent meals to ease digestion and reduce gas buildup.

3. **Chew Food Thoroughly:**
   - Properly chewing your food helps break it down more effectively, which can minimize gas formation. Take your time to chew each bite well.

4. **Stay Hydrated:**
   - Drinking plenty of fluids, especially water, helps move food through your digestive system and can reduce gas.

5. **Try Simethicone:**

- Over-the-counter medications containing simethicone can help reduce gas and bloating. Consult with your healthcare provider before using any new medication.

**Managing Odor**

1. **Choose Odor-Reducing Foods:**
   - Some foods are less likely to cause odor, including lean proteins, white rice, and plain yogurt. Incorporate these into your diet to help manage odor.

2. **Use Odor-Controlling Products:**
   - Specialized deodorizing products are available for ostomy bags. Consider using deodorizing drops or filters designed to neutralize odors.

3. **Maintain Good Hygiene:**
   - Regularly clean the skin around your stoma and the inside of your ostomy bag. Keeping the area clean can help reduce unpleasant odors.

4. **Ventilation:**
   - Ensure that your ostomy bag is not overly full. An overfilled bag can lead to more noticeable odors. Empty it regularly.

5. **Avoid Foods That Increase Odor:**
   - Foods such as onions, garlic, and certain spices can increase odor. Be mindful of these when planning your meals.

**Managing Stool Consistency**

1. **Monitor Your Diet:**
   - Eating a balanced diet with the right consistency of foods can help manage stool consistency. Opt for low-fiber foods that are easier to digest.

2. **Increase or Decrease Fiber Intake Gradually:**
   - While high-fiber foods are generally more challenging, certain soluble fibers can help regulate stool consistency. Introduce these slowly and observe how your body responds.

3. **Stay Hydrated:**

- Adequate fluid intake is essential for maintaining the right stool consistency. Aim to drink plenty of fluids throughout the day.

4. **Use Thickening Agents:**
   - If you experience very loose stool, consider using thickening agents like soluble fiber supplements or pectin, with guidance from your healthcare provider.

5. **Consult Your Healthcare Provider:**
   - If you encounter persistent issues with stool consistency, seek advice from your healthcare provider. They can provide personalized recommendations and adjustments to your diet or treatment plan.

## *What to Do If You Experience Blockages or Discomfort*

Experiencing blockages or discomfort can be a common concern for individuals with a colostomy or ileostomy. Understanding how to manage these situations effectively is crucial for maintaining your well-being and preventing complications. Here's a guide on what to do if you encounter blockages or discomfort:

**Managing Blockages**

1. **Recognize the Symptoms:**
   - Symptoms of a blockage can include cramping, abdominal pain, swelling, nausea, vomiting, or a reduction in the output from your ostomy bag. If you experience any of these signs, it's important to act promptly.

2. **Stay Hydrated:**
   - Drink plenty of fluids to help move the blockage through your digestive system. Water and clear broths are excellent choices. Avoid carbonated beverages, as they can worsen bloating.

3. **Gently Massage Your Abdomen:**
   - Lightly massaging your abdomen can sometimes help relieve mild blockages. Use gentle, circular motions to encourage movement in your digestive tract.

4. **Try the "Knee-Chest" Position:**

- Getting into the knee-chest position—kneeling and bringing your chest to your knees—can sometimes help relieve a blockage by applying pressure to your abdomen.

5. **Avoid Certain Foods:**

    - If you suspect a blockage, avoid foods that are known to cause obstructions, such as nuts, seeds, popcorn, and certain fibrous vegetables.

6. **Consult Your Healthcare Provider:**

    - If symptoms persist or worsen despite these measures, contact your healthcare provider. They can provide further guidance and, if necessary, perform an examination to address the blockage.

7. **Consider an Enema:**

    - In some cases, your healthcare provider might recommend using a gentle enema to help clear the blockage. Only use enemas under medical supervision.

**Managing Discomfort**

1. **Identify the Source:**

    - Determine whether the discomfort is related to your stoma, surrounding skin, or internal issues. Understanding the source can help in addressing the problem effectively.

2. **Check Your Ostomy Equipment:**

    - Ensure that your ostomy bag and skin barrier are properly fitted and secure. Leaks or improper fitting can cause irritation and discomfort.

3. **Use Barrier Creams or Sprays:**

    - Applying a barrier cream or spray can help protect the skin around your stoma from irritation. Choose products specifically designed for ostomy care.

4. **Adjust Your Diet:**

    - Certain foods can cause discomfort or irritation. If you notice a pattern, consider adjusting your diet to avoid those specific foods. Opt for bland, low-fiber foods if you're experiencing discomfort.

5. **Take Over-the-Counter Pain Relief:**
    - For mild discomfort, over-the-counter pain relievers like acetaminophen or ibuprofen may be helpful. Always follow the dosage instructions and consult your healthcare provider before taking any new medication.

6. **Wear Loose Clothing:**
    - Tight clothing can exacerbate discomfort. Opt for loose, comfortable clothing that doesn't put pressure on your stoma or abdomen.

7. **Seek Professional Advice:**
    - If discomfort is severe or persistent, seek advice from your healthcare provider. They can offer solutions, such as adjusting your ostomy equipment or exploring other treatment options.

## *Strategies for Dining Out and Social Situations*

Navigating dining out and social situations with a colostomy or ileostomy can pose unique challenges. However, with the right strategies, you can enjoy meals and social gatherings with confidence and comfort. Here's how to manage dining out and social situations effectively:

**1. Plan Ahead**

- **Research Restaurants:** Before heading out, check the restaurant's menu online to identify suitable options. Many restaurants now offer allergen and ingredient information, which can be helpful in making informed choices.
- **Call Ahead:** If you have specific dietary needs or restrictions, consider calling the restaurant in advance to discuss your options. Most establishments are willing to accommodate special requests.

**2. Choose Your Foods Wisely**

- **Opt for Low-Fiber Foods:** Select dishes that are low in fiber and easy to digest, such as well-cooked lean meats, white rice, and plain pasta. Avoid foods known to cause gas or discomfort, such as beans, cruciferous vegetables, and high-fat items.
- **Avoid High-Risk Foods:** Steer clear of foods that may lead to blockages or discomfort, such as raw vegetables, nuts, and foods with tough skins or seeds.

### 3. Manage Your Stoma and Equipment

- **Carry Essentials:** Bring along extra ostomy supplies, such as bags and skin barriers, to ensure you're prepared for any situation. Consider carrying a small, discreet pouch with your essentials.

- **Empty Before You Go:** To minimize the risk of leaks or discomfort, empty your ostomy bag before leaving for your meal. This also helps you feel more comfortable and confident.

### 4. Communicate Your Needs

- **Be Open with Your Host:** If attending a social event, inform your host about any special dietary needs or restrictions. Most people are understanding and willing to accommodate dietary concerns.

- **Request Modifications:** Don't hesitate to ask for modifications to dishes when dining out. For example, you can request that your food be prepared without certain ingredients or that it be cooked in a specific way.

### 5. Be Mindful of Your Comfort

- **Choose Comfortable Seating:** Select a seat that allows you to feel relaxed and at ease. Avoid tight spaces or positions that might put pressure on your stoma.

- **Plan Breaks:** If you anticipate needing a break during the meal, plan ahead to find a convenient time for restroom breaks or adjustments.

### 6. Practice Discretion

- **Be Confident:** Remember that having an ostomy is a part of who you are, but it doesn't define you. Approach social situations with confidence and focus on enjoying your time with others.

- **Carry a Discreet Bag:** Use a discreet, odor-proof bag to manage any potential issues. Many options are designed to be inconspicuous and easy to carry.

### 7. Addressing Emergencies

- **Know Your Facilities:** Familiarize yourself with the location of restrooms and facilities in restaurants or social venues. This can help you feel more prepared and reduce anxiety.

- **Stay Calm:** If an unexpected situation arises, such as a leak or discomfort, remain calm and address it as needed. Most people are understanding, and you can always excuse yourself briefly if necessary.

8. **Enjoy the Moment**

    - **Focus on the Experience:** Dining out and socializing are about enjoying good company and experiences. Don't let concerns about your ostomy overshadow the pleasure of the occasion.

    - **Share Your Journey:** If you feel comfortable, sharing your experiences with friends and family can foster understanding and support, making social situations more enjoyable for everyone.

# Chapter 15

# FAQs and Troubleshooting

**What are the 4 sites for a colostomy?**

The four common sites for a colostomy are:

1. **Ascending Colon (Right Side):** This site is used for a colostomy where the stoma is located on the right side of the abdomen. It usually produces liquid stool.

2. **Transverse Colon (Middle):** This colostomy is placed across the upper abdomen and may produce semi-formed stool.

3. **Descending Colon (Left Side):** The stoma is on the left side of the abdomen, and the stool is usually more formed.

4. **Sigmoid Colon (Lower Left Side):** This site is often used for a colostomy that results in well-formed stool.

**What are the 4 types of colostomies?**

1. **End Colostomy:** The end of the colon is brought through the abdominal wall to create a stoma. It may be permanent or temporary.

2. **Loop Colostomy:** A loop of the colon is brought to the surface, and both ends of the loop are attached to the abdominal wall. This type is usually temporary.

3. **Double-Barrel Colostomy:** The colon is divided, and both ends are brought to the abdominal wall as two separate stomas. This is typically temporary.

4. **Hartmann's Procedure:** A part of the colon is removed, and the remaining part is brought out as a stoma. The remaining part of the bowel is usually left to heal.

**Which organ is removed during a colostomy?**

During a colostomy, a portion of the colon (large intestine) is removed or bypassed, depending on the type and reason for the surgery. The rectum and potentially part of the sigmoid colon may also be removed or bypassed.

**What is the biggest patient problem for a colostomy?**

One of the biggest challenges for colostomy patients is managing stool consistency and odor, as well as preventing skin irritation and maintaining a proper fit of the colostomy pouch. Psychological and emotional adjustment to the ostomy can also be significant concerns.

**When Should I Change My Colostomy Pouch?**

You should change your colostomy pouch when it is full, when the adhesive starts to peel away, or if there is any leakage or irritation around the stoma. Regular checks will help maintain skin health and pouch effectiveness.

**How Should I Care for the Stomal Area?**

- **Clean Gently:** Use mild soap and water to clean around the stoma, avoiding harsh chemicals.
- **Dry Thoroughly:** Make sure the area is completely dry before applying a new pouch to prevent skin irritation.
- **Inspect Regularly:** Check for any signs of irritation, infection, or unusual changes in the stoma.

**How Should I Bathe with a Colostomy?**

You can bathe or shower with your colostomy pouch on or off, depending on your comfort level. Ensure the pouch is securely fastened if you choose to keep it on, and use mild, non-irritating soap and water.

**How Should I Exercise with a Colostomy?**

- **Start Slowly:** Begin with gentle exercises and gradually increase intensity as you build confidence.
- **Choose Low-Impact Activities:** Activities like walking, swimming, and cycling are generally safe.
- **Secure the Pouch:** Use a support belt or cover to keep the pouch in place during exercise.

**Will Weight Gain or Loss Affect My Colostomy Pouch?**

Yes, significant weight changes can affect the fit of your colostomy pouch. Regularly monitor your weight and adjust the size or type of pouch as needed. Consult with your healthcare provider for recommendations.

**What Are Some Other Helpful Tips for a Colostomy?**

- **Stay Hydrated**: Drink plenty of fluids to prevent dehydration.
- **Maintain a Balanced Diet**: Follow dietary recommendations to manage stool consistency.
- **Keep a Stoma Diary**: Track changes in your stoma and stool to identify patterns and issues.

**How Should I Travel with a Colostomy Pouch?**

- **Pack Supplies**: Bring extra pouches, adhesive products, and cleaning materials.
- **Plan**: Know the location of restrooms and facilities.
- **Keep Pouches Secure**: Use travel-sized containers and ensure pouches are securely packed.

**Tips to Help with Your Ostomy**

- **Be Patient**: Give yourself time to adjust to your ostomy and find what works best for you.
- **Seek Support**: Join support groups or talk to others who have experienced similar challenges.

**When Should I Call the ET Nurse?**

Call your Enterostomal Therapy (ET) nurse if you experience:

- **Skin Irritation**: Persistent redness or breakdown around the stoma.
- **Stoma Changes**: Significant changes in size, color, or output.
- **Pouch Issues**: Frequent leaks or difficulties with pouch adhesion.

**How many times do you empty your pouch in one day? How do you empty it?**

The frequency of emptying your pouch can vary, but it's typically done 3 to 5 times a day. To empty it, open the bottom of the pouch, and pour the contents into the toilet. Clean the pouch as needed and securely close it afterward.

**What can you eat with an ostomy?**

Focus on low-fiber, well-cooked foods that are easy to digest, such as white rice, cooked chicken, and peeled fruits. Avoid high-fiber and gas-producing foods until you understand how they affect your stoma.

**Can you control your bowel movements?**

With a colostomy, you cannot control bowel movements as you would with a normal colon. The output is collected in the pouch, and you manage it by changing the pouch as needed.

**What can I do to eliminate or lessen odor?**

- **Use Odor-Control Products:** Specialized sprays or filters can help manage odor.
- **Choose Foods Wisely:** Avoid foods known to cause strong odors.
- **Keep the Pouch Clean:** Regular cleaning and proper pouch fitting help reduce odor.

**Can you get in the water?**

Yes, you can swim and bathe with a colostomy. Ensure your pouch is securely attached and consider using waterproof covers if needed.

**What clothes can you wear with an ostomy?**

Wear comfortable, loose-fitting clothing. Avoid tight belts or clothing that may put pressure on your stoma. Many people find that high-waisted or adjustable clothing works best.

**Can you have an intimate relationship or get pregnant with an ostomy?**

Yes, having an ostomy does not prevent you from having an intimate relationship or getting pregnant. Communicate openly with your partner and consult with your healthcare provider about any concerns.

**How do you tell people about your ostomy?**

You can choose to share your ostomy information as you feel comfortable. Being open and educating others can help foster understanding and support.

**How do I care for my new colostomy after ostomy surgery?**

- **Follow Care Instructions:** Adhere to your healthcare provider's guidelines for pouch care and skin maintenance.

- **Monitor for Issues:** Watch for signs of infection, irritation, or other complications.

- **Attend Follow-Up Appointments:** Regular check-ups ensure your ostomy is functioning well and provide opportunities to address any concerns.

**How will living with a colostomy affect my life?**

Living with a colostomy may require adjustments in diet, lifestyle, and personal routines. However, with proper care and support, many people lead active, fulfilling lives.

**Will I have to change my diet after colostomy surgery?**

Yes, you may need to modify your diet to manage stool consistency and minimize discomfort. Focus on low-fiber, easily digestible foods and introduce new foods gradually.

**What does a stoma look like?**

A stoma is a small, round, reddish-pink protrusion on the abdomen where the colon or ileum is attached. It should be moist and healthy-looking, with no signs of significant discoloration or swelling.

# Conclusion

Your ostomy is a part of your life, but it does not dictate the limits of your experiences or the joy you can find in each day. Embracing life with confidence is about acknowledging your strength and resilience and recognizing that you have the power to adapt and thrive.

Adjusting to life with an ostomy can present challenges, but it also offers an opportunity for personal growth and empowerment. This cookbook is designed to support you in making this transition as smooth as possible by providing practical, delicious, and easy-to-digest recipes tailored for your needs. Whether you are just starting your ostomy journey or have been living with one for some time, the right food can play a crucial role in managing your health and enhancing your quality of life.

Remember, you do not have to navigate this journey alone. Lean on the support of family, friends, and healthcare professionals. Use the knowledge and tools you have gained to build a routine that works best for you. Every small step you take towards understanding your body's needs and preferences is a victory.

**Final Thoughts and Encouragement**

Living with an ostomy is a testament to your resilience and adaptability. It's a journey that requires patience, self-care, and a willingness to explore new ways of living. Embrace the changes with an open heart and a positive outlook. You can lead a fulfilling life, enjoy delicious meals, and participate fully in activities you love.

This cookbook is more than just a collection of recipes—it is a guide to help you nourish your body, enjoy your meals, and feel confident in your daily life. Each recipe has been crafted with care to ensure it supports your digestive health while providing the satisfaction of great taste.

As you move forward, remember that your ostomy is just one part of who you are. Embrace the opportunities that lie ahead and know that you have the strength to overcome any obstacles. Your journey is unique, and with the right support and resources, you can embrace life with confidence and joy.

Thank you for allowing this cookbook to be a part of your journey. Here is to a future filled with health, happiness, and the confidence to live your life to the fullest.

Made in the USA
Las Vegas, NV
27 June 2025